Stella's Story: Fighting for Life Against a Malignant Brain Tumor

Stella's Story: Fighting for Life Against a Malignant Brain Tumor

Kay Loveland

iUniverse, Inc.
New York Lincoln Shanghai

Stella's Story: Fighting for Life Against a Malignant Brain Tumor

iUniverse, Inc.

For information address:
iUniverse, Inc.
2021 Pine Lake Road, Suite 100
Lincoln, NE 68512
www.iuniverse.com

ISBN: 0-595-31960-2

Printed in the United States of America

Contents

Introduction vii

Section 1. The First Nine Months. 1

Covers first symptoms, diagnosis, first craniotomy, standard radiation, seizure, second craniotomy, in-patient and out-patient rehabilitation, exploration of chemotherapy and other treatments, stereotactic radiosurgery, beginnings of Stella's downhill slide

Section 2. The Next Six Months 46

Covers stable tumor throughout this period, chemotherapy (CCNU & Temodar), Stella's increasing loss of cognitive and physical functions and Kay's search for answers, in-patient rehabilitation in nursing home and at National Rehabilitation Hospital, decision to take Stella to Mexican clinic for vaccine & holistic therapies, seven-week stay in Mexico, question of hydrocephalus, first mention by a doctor of delayed radiation injury as cause of Stella's six-month decline resulting in her inability to function in any way by late June

Section 3. The Last Five Months. 124

Covers efforts to get opinions from doctors and research into whether Stella was suffering from normal-pressure hydrocephalus and/or radiation injury and whether a shunt might help her regain some functioning, numerous hospitalizations for tests, infections, shunt surgery, communications with UCLA center specializing in adult hydrocephalus, research on medications (Ritalin, Provigil, bromocriptine, L-Dopa and other Parkinson's and Alzheimer's drugs) that might increase Stella's alertness and functioning, search for a local doctor who could (and would) administer such medications, exploration of taking Stella to Duke or UCLA brain tumor centers for comprehensive evaluation and treatment, efforts to get doctors to prescribe chemotherapy for Stella, first MRI showing regrowth of tumor since December, exploration of whether a team specializing in work with coma patients might help Stella, Stella's death.

Index. 219

Introduction

The nightmare began on April 21, 1999. My partner of thirty years, Stella (Stel) Sandris, was in a lunch meeting at the National Gallery of Art in Washington, D.C., excitedly discussing a lecture-film proposal she had made to the Gallery. She suddenly felt numbness in her left arm and hand, dizziness, and nausea. She thought she was having a stroke. Not wanting to upset the others at the table, she managed to get through the meeting without anyone suspecting how she was feeling. She left the Gallery, walked a few blocks to the Metro (subway) stop, rode back to where she had parked the car, and drove several miles back to our apartment in Bethesda, Maryland, all the while fighting off the sense that she was going to pass out. When she got home, she called me at my office.

I had happily awaited her phone call, expecting to hear that she had had a wonderful lunch with her friends and colleagues at the Gallery. It was approaching 5:00 and I was a little perplexed as to why I hadn't heard from her when the phone rang. I quickly answered it and immediately said, "Hi sweetheart, how was your—". Stel interrupted my question. "I'm feeling very ill," she said. She spoke calmly, explaining to me what had happened and how she felt. I automatically chastised her for not telling her friends at lunch and for not calling me instead of taking the risk of driving herself all the way home. At the same time, my mind was racing off in different directions: This couldn't be that serious. Could it be a heart attack? Surely not. Stel had just had a full physical, including a treadmill test, two months before that she passed with flying colors. In all the years I had known her, she had never suffered from more than an occasional cold. She had never been in the hospital in her life. I had told her more than once that she was one of the healthiest people I had ever known. She ate properly, didn't smoke, drank moderately. There had been a disproportionate number of grave illnesses and deaths in the younger members of her family in recent years; I thought the odds must be with her. Yet, at the same time, I was frightened because I knew Stel wouldn't tell me she was "feeling very ill" unless she thought it was serious. I said she should go to the emergency room at a hospital a few minutes from our apartment. She insisted she could drive herself there. In my most emphatic voice, I said, "No you can't. Stay where you are, and I'll be right there."

I quickly gathered up my things, told a colleague I had an emergency at home and asked if he could take over for me the next day, if necessary, in supervising the taping of a TV program I was responsible for (adding that I thought everything would be okay and I would be at work tomorrow), and dashed to the Metro. All the way home, I kept going over in my mind all the reasons why Stel couldn't be seriously ill, trying to remember any incidents in recent weeks that might give me a clue as to what was going on.[1] I just could not imagine my healthy, vibrant Stella being sick for more than a couple of days. I had every expectation and happy anticipation that we would add another fifteen or twenty years to the almost thirty we had already spent together.

When the train got to my home stop, I ran out of the station and hailed a cab for the two-minute ride to the apartment (Stel picked me up most days). I found her sitting on the bed. She said she was feeling better and maybe she didn't need to go to the emergency room. "Yes you do," I said, as I pulled her off the bed. We walked down the long hall to our front door, down the ten steps that led outside, and out to the car parked thirty steps or so from the front entrance. Stel seemed perfectly normal. The drive was less than ten minutes to the hospital. I pulled into a parking space in front of the ER and took Stella's hand as we walked toward the door. "Hold me up, Kate," she said quietly as we approached the entrance, "My leg feels spongy." We checked her in and they took her into the

---

1. After we learned a few days later that she had a brain tumor, I looked back on several occurrences over the last year or so that I realized probably were tumor-related. In the weeks before going to the emergency room, we thought Stel was having sinus problems because of pain she was experiencing on the right side of her face. We believed this was related to the only surgery she had ever had and that she had long regretted—an out-patient procedure 25 years before to alleviate a sinus condition. The operation had not accomplished what had been promised and had left her face in that area overly sensitive. Also, on a few occasions, Stel had dropped almost instantaneously into a deep, black depression that was uncharacteristic of her, but at the time I felt there were external reasons why she could be feeling so despairing in those moments. I also felt she was more nervous and anxious than usual, but attributed that to external factors as well, particularly exhaustion from months of intense activity. It seemed to me, as well, that she was having more difficulty than usual in organizing her writing—repeating things, leaving some sentences unfinished—but again I thought it probably resulted from the exhausting schedule she faced in meeting multiple deadlines in a brief time. It was unusal, too, that she was sleeping later in the mornings since she had always been an early riser. All of these, I came to believe, were at least partially manifestations of the tumor.

ER, telling me I could join her in a few minutes. When they finally let me go in, she had had a CT scan and her blood had been taken for tests. They had given her medication for nausea and dizziness. I sat at her bedside for six hours as we watched all of the commotion in the ER with new cases arriving and wondered, as time dragged on and all the doctors and nurses seemed oblivious to us, whether Stel had been forgotten in the frenetic activity. At one point, a nurse came in to ask her how she was feeling; Stel responded that she felt fine; the numbness, nausea and dizziness had ceased. My heart lifted when the nurse said that was good and probably indicated that the inner ear was the cause of Stel's problems. "Yes," I said to myself with relief. "That must be the reason." I was more convinced of it as various test results came back negative and allowed myself to believe that they would soon pronounce Stel okay to go home and not to worry. I don't remember what she and I said to each other during those long hours. I know she was relieved that she was no longer feeling ill and I'm sure she was cheered by the nurse's words.

Also running through my mind during those hours was the surreal contrast between this night spent in the ER and the night before when Stel had taught a five-hour documentary film class at American University. She had prepared meticulously for it for several weeks, discussing intensely with me the film clips she wanted to show and the reading material she wanted the class to have. All of her work had come to fruition after the class, when many students came up to tell her how interesting and stimulating they had found her presentation. I was there, not only because, as always, I was interested in what she had to say but also, as always, to help her however I could. I was in charge of playing the film clips she interspersed with her lecture. It had been a very happy evening and we celebrated with a drink and talked animatedly about future projects before going home. Then whammo! Less than twenty-four hours later, Stella lay in the ER, and I felt our happiness of the night before mocked by the fear and anxiety now fluttering in my mind. For the first, but certainly not the last, time in the nineteen-month ordeal we were unknowingly entering upon, I felt as if I had been sideswiped.

Finally, about midnight, the doctor came quickly into Stella's cubicle. He was agitated. He asked for the name and phone number of her internist and then said to Stel that the CT scan showed "a mass on the brain." My heart jumped into my throat; I probably stood with my mouth gaping. The thought of a brain tumor had never entered my mind and I had been so reassured by the good results of all the other tests that I really had convinced myself he would tell Stel it was nothing to worry about. I couldn't believe my ears. He told her they couldn't tell from the scan what "the mass" was and she should have an MRI the next day, which he would ask her internist to arrange. I remember him saying he didn't want to be "doom and gloom, but"—whatever he said after that, and the look of dread on his face, conveyed that he was, if not "gloomy," at least very apprehensive about what "the mass" was. He asked Stel if any members of her family had had brain tumors. She said "no," apparently thinking only of her immediate family or perhaps wanting to forget that her niece had died of a Grade IV tumor almost twelve years before. I immediately thought of her niece and felt fear spike up in my heart. (Looking back, knowing as I do now that there is no solid scientific evidence that brain tumors run in families, I see his question as typical of the lack of knowledge about them that we encountered among many doctors.) God knows what emotions and thoughts were coursing through Stel's mind during those moments. She gave no outward sign of shock or fear. After the doctor left to call her internist, I helped her get off the gurney and put her clothes on. In the midst of it, tears began to roll down my cheeks. Stella said gently but firmly, "Don't cry, Kate." I responded, "I can't help it." She was soon discharged with medication for nausea and dizziness and instructions to call her internist in the morning to find out when the MRI was scheduled. And so around midnight, we drove back to the apartment having no idea what terrors and heartaches lay ahead, not yet understanding fully that our lives had changed forever. For the next nineteen months we would fight for her life against the deadliest of tumors—glioblastoma multiforme (GBM), a Grade IV brain tumor in her right frontal lobe just in front of the motor strip that ultimately crossed over to the left hemisphere through the corpus callosum.

In those months, Stella underwent two craniotomies within three months (due to the first surgeon's failures), six and one-half weeks of standard radiation, seven weeks of in-patient physical, occupational and speech therapy, six weeks of at-home therapy, four weeks of out-patient therapy, one-shot stereotactic radiosurgery, three rounds of chemotherapy, seven weeks of alternative treatment in Mexico, surgery for placement of a shunt, and spent at least eighteen weeks in hospitals and clinics and seven weeks in nursing homes. This very healthy woman who rarely and reluctantly took drugs of any kind, including aspirin, was subjected to round-upon-round of medications meant to prevent seizures (Dilantin, Tegretol, Depakote), decrease brain swelling (Decadron), stop nausea (Zofran and others), protect her stomach from the effects of other medicines (Prevacid, Zantac), fight depression (Paxil), kill the tumor (CCNU, Temodar), increase alertness (Ritalin, bromocriptine, Provigil and others), and fight infections (various antibiotics). There were undoubtedly many others that don't come readily to mind. In addition, she had vaccine shots in Mexico, and throughout her illness took myriad supplements to boost her immune system, fight the tumor, and bolster her body and health in a variety of ways.

I was at her side day-in and day-out through all of the doctors' appointments, surgeries, treatments, hospitalizations, and nursing-home stays. I hated it that I couldn't be with her in the operating rooms and radiation chambers, the most terrifying places of all. For eight weeks after Stel's first surgery on May 6, 1999, I was able to work about twenty hours at my office and fifteen hours at home, but after her second surgery on August 10, 1999, I didn't enter the door of my office again until January 16, 2001, two months after she died. I was fortunate to be a federal government employee who could receive donated annual leave from other federal employees throughout the country when mine ran out and, for that reason, was able to hang onto my job even though I couldn't do any work at all for about fourteen months (aside from the initial eight weeks mentioned above, I managed to do part-time work at home editing a book from July to October 2000). I couldn't take advantage of the Family and Medical Leave Act (the entitlement to three months of leave without pay to take care of a seriously ill family member) because my partnership of thirty years with a woman was not recognized by that law. However, I was relieved to find out that Stel was considered my family under the Family Friendly Leave Act, and I was able to use a total of about five weeks of accumulated sick leave to care for her.[2] Without those benefits and the financial assistance of some good friends (our families were either unwilling or unable to offer help financially and, for the most part, personally), I not only would have lost my beloved friend and companion to this horrendous illness but also my livelihood and most of whatever financial reserves we had been able to amass for retirement. At the age of 60 (my birthday was a week after Stella died), I would have confronted financial ruin while trying to deal with the greatest emotional loss of my life.

Like most brain tumor patients and their caregivers, Stella and I underwent a crash course in brain tumors during those first dreadfully frightening days and weeks from the night in the ER to our first meeting with her neurosurgeon five days later to her first craniotomy just fifteen days after learning she had a "mass on her brain" to the beginning of her radiation treatment four weeks after sur-

---

2.   The law allows employees to use up to as much as twelve weeks of accumulated sick leave to care for family members.

gery. By then we knew the devastating prognosis that even with surgery and radiation, the median survival of GBM patients was about ten months; we were not clear at all about whether chemotherapy could be effective but were being steered by the oncologist Stel's neurosurgeon had referred her to toward PCV starting several weeks after radiation. We knew next to nothing about other chemo options or any other forms of therapy including stereotactic radiosurgery. While Stel was undergoing radiation, I commissioned a report from The Health Resource, a medical information service (800-949-0090; www. thehealthresource.com), about treatments for GBMs which provided me with more information about these mainstream options as well as some non-mainstream treatments. I also got a report on alternative treatments from well-known researcher Ralph Moss, Ph.D. (800-980-1234; www.ralphmoss.com). I had also found the book Choices in Healing by Michael Lerner, a general book about cancer, which I found informative and helpful in beginning to understand the choices we would have to confront among conventional and alternative therapies. There were other books and articles dealing with cancer that I got my hands on, and a friend helped me get a list of clinical trials and other information on brain tumors from the National Cancer Institute. The information we had and where it came from at that point is pretty hazy in my mind now, but I know Stel and I weren't fully convinced that PCV was the way to go after radiation and were searching for other answers. I did not discover the Brain Tumor List (Listserv@mitvma.mit.edu) and the Virtual Trials website (http:// virtualtrials.com) until after Stella's second surgery. When I did, they became great sources of information about standard and new mainstream treatments and, especially, about what patients and caregivers were experiencing on a daily basis. And I read there of several people with GBMs who were outliving by years their terminal prognosis. I told Stella about them and voiced my belief that she could do that, too.

Sometime in the midst of those frantic weeks of trying to learn as much as possible as quickly as possible about a horrifying and sickening subject, it began to dawn on me that the medical profession knew very little about the brain in general and brain tumors—especially GBMs—in particular. That night back in the ER I had thought of Stella's niece who had died in 1987 and said to myself, "but that was twelve years ago; they're bound to have made a lot of progress since then." What I learned to my increasing alarm was that hardly anything had changed in the treatment of GBMs in twenty-five years. The chemos the oncologist had mentioned—BCNU, PCV—had been used for years, and they were effective for only a minority of patients. In light of this, I also began to realize that an attitude of extreme pessimism, even nihilism, pervaded much of the medical profession with regard to GBM patients. To many doctors outside of the national brain tumor centers, a GBM patient is, for all practical purposes, already dead, and patients and caregivers who persist in fighting to beat the miserable odds are hopelessly deluded. Several doctors at one time or another essentially told me I was crazy to think that anyone survived a GBM. They just discounted the experiences of the long-term survivors I knew of on the BT List as people whose diagnoses must have been wrong, or who must have misunderstood their diagnoses. I'm sure that Stel, who was an extremely perceptive and sensitive person, was aware of this attitude, but we never talked about it to each other. I always tried to counter such pessimism with what I knew about patients who were surviving and emphasized the reasons she could be one of them—her healthy body ("a perfect specimen of health," the oncologist had said, "except for the tumor"); her youthfulness (Stel was 59 when she was diagnosed but in every way was at least ten years younger; I knew the bad odds grew worse with age but believed Stel didn't fit in the older category); the small size of the tumor (2 cm) when it was diagnosed; her strength in coming through surgery and radiation; her fighting spirit.

There are many deeply frustrating and depressing situations and problems that brain tumor patients and their caregivers must deal with, but I believe trying to cope with the profound pessimism of so many doctors is among the most difficult. These doctors simply don't seem to understand that most of us need some sense of hope in order to confront on a daily basis the terrors and horrors of such an insidious disease. (I should distinguish here between the local doctors we dealt with, for whom brain tumors are only a small part of their practice, from doctors at brain tumor centers who treat nothing else. Perhaps because they see the full range of experiences of BT patients and actually treat people who defy their grim prognoses, these doctors usually convey a more hopeful attitude. If I had realized this sooner, I would have raised heaven and earth to move Stel to a city with a BT center for continuing treatment.[3]) Perhaps there is a small minority of patients who, when told they have an aggressive tumor devouring their brain and a life expectancy of a few months, can say, "Okay. Since there's no hope, I'm going to go home and enjoy myself and my loved ones for the time I have." But we didn't

---

3.   I want to acknowledge particularly Drs. Christina Meyers at M.D. Anderson, Henry Friedman at Duke University, and Alejandro Torres-Trejo who was at UCLA at that time.

encounter any people like that on our BT journey. Like Stella and me, they wanted to fight, wanted to hope that, however great the odds, they (we) might prevail. That glimmer of hope gave life enough meaning to sustain us, even in the face of unbearable tragedy. The doctors who allowed no hope, who discounted the possibility that there were some people who were outliving their prognoses, who spoke as if we were foolishly naive to think Stel might have any chance of winning this battle, needlessly added more agony to lives already lived on the edge of despair.

In some of my e-mails included in this book I spoke of my struggle to keep the doctors' pessimism from killing Stella, and I meant that literally. Because of the very negative attitudes of many doctors toward GBM patients, they are often unwilling to consider, let alone try, new or alternative treatments. In their eyes, it is pointless to expend more energy and money on patients who are as good as dead already. (Undoubtedly, many of them feel that it is wrong and perhaps unethical to offer even the slightest encouragement, which they consider false hope. I've already voiced above my feeling about the importance of allowing patients to have some hope, however slim.) Very quickly, they begin pushing caregivers and families toward hospice, frequently in the patient's presence. I was furious when different doctors did this in front of Stel on several occasions and immediately cut them off in mid-sentence. The constant fight against this negativity drained energy I needed for dealing with all the other obstacles that confronted us and consequently made life that much harder.

The unwelcome education of BT patients and caregivers, thrust with little or no warning into a surreal, terrifying world, takes place in the midst of a frantic, roller-coaster existence. We must learn as fast as we can because, for many of these tumors—and especially a GBM—we know we're in a race against time. We find out very soon how little the medical profession really knows and how inadequate the conventional treatments are; and once past surgery and standard radiation, we realize that the choice of treatments—a life and death matter—is completely a crapshoot. Later, some of us learn—as I did with Stella—to our great dismay that the effects of standard radiation treatment, which supposedly delivers the maximum "safe" dose to the brain, can be far more devastating than we ever could have imagined when our doctors quickly rattled off the possible consequences back in those early, dazed weeks following surgery and diagnosis. Fortunately, the Internet has opened up avenues of information and education that didn't exist for brain tumor patients a few years ago, and I'm very grateful for having had access to the Brain Tumor List and the Musella Virtual Trials website, in particular, through which I learned a great deal about the disease that had invaded our lives and the pros and cons of a variety of treatments for it. Equally important, I found invaluable advice, understanding, and support that helped me survive bleak and lonely times.

Having come through trial by torture and terror (which, I am sure, will inhabit my heart and soul for the rest of my life), I looked back at that nightmarish descent into the abyss and wished I had had a sort of guidebook to alert me to the unimaginable number of obstacles and experiences Stel and I might face on that journey. In the early days of Stella's illness, I read a couple of books by survivors or caregivers that dealt in fairly broad strokes with what they had experienced, but there was nothing that really chronicled the day-to-day struggle. In 2002, an excellent book by Ben Williams, Surviving 'Terminal' Cancer, was published. Professor Williams, in his late fifties or early sixties, is one of the long-time survivors of a GBM whom I first read about on the Musella website and whose story gave us hope. He writes about receiving a death sentence in 1995 and the treatments he devised mostly by himself that have proven successful thus far in vanquishing the tumor. It is a book I urge every patient and caregiver, and every neurosurgeon and oncologist, to read. It is not, however, a daily chronicle of what one may face and the decisions one may have to make in the, unfortunately, more typical experience of GBM patients and caregivers. Reading the messages on the Brain Tumor List every day does give one a sense of that but, by its nature, the List is fragmented and it's difficult (and time-consuming) to go back through an archive of thousands of messages (the list averaged about 100 a day in the fifteen months or so when I was reading it religiously) to gain the sense of continuity and history that a book can provide.

In light of everything Stella and I went through, I felt I had important knowledge and experience that might be helpful to others in similar circumstances, and I wanted to write a narrative that would give a sense to those who read it of what they might encounter on the road ahead. (I should emphasize that a defining characteristic of the disease is its unpredictability. In that sense, Stel's story is unique and, indeed, her case was unusual, even in the GBM universe, because for nine months her tumor didn't grow while at the same time, she lost her ability to function completely. To my heartbreak, she experienced for a very long period of time what many BT patients experience only in the last days or weeks of their illness. Nevertheless, patients and caregivers must deal with many of the same problems and obstacles that we did in the course of the illness and, unfortunately, they can't predict what unusual twists and turns the road may take. Consequently, I believe this chronicle of what we coped with can provide much helpful information to most people who must travel through the same unknown terrain.) As I looked through the hundreds of e-mails I wrote to and received from friends, relatives, Brain Tumor List members, doctors, and others during those harrowing months, I realized that the story was already written and it was a matter of culling and editing the messages to provide the clearest account possible of our struggle. And that is what I've tried to do in this book. Through the e-mails and the daily journal I kept during the seven weeks we were in Mexico, readers can follow our journey nearly every step of the way. (For privacy reasons, I've changed the names of patients and caregivers.) It begins twenty-six days before we had any inkling of the catastrophe about to strike us with e-mails written by Stel, her friends and co-workers, and me and ends almost twenty months later, two days after Stella's death. It is not easy reading; nothing one reads about this horrendous disease is. But for those who want to have some idea of what may lie ahead, it can alert them to many of the decisions, hurdles and unexpected occurrences they may have to confront. I feel sure that if such a chronicle had been available to me, I would have found such help in it and not only would not have felt blindsided so often by events, but might have been armed sooner with knowledge that would have enabled me to take action—such as moving Stella immediately to a location with a national brain tumor center for ongoing treatment—that might have had a significant impact on the quality, and perhaps the quantity, of her life.

Putting this book together has been a painful endeavor as I've relived so many heartrending moments and been reminded of the impossible, gut-wrenching decisions that confronted me and the deeply frustrating interactions I had with medical professionals, insurance personnel, and others. But there were moments of joy in it, too, as I experienced again those all-too-brief times when the lively, articulate, warm Stella I knew so well "came back" and my heart leapt up in hope that this might portend the beginning of a new day. (I also rediscovered moments of happiness that had been buried under memories of unrelenting sadness. If I hadn't written about them at the time, I fear they would have been lost to me forever.) It was a roller-coaster ride emotionally—one it is hard to imagine unless you have lived it—and when I began reading the e-mail archive I had accumulated over twenty months, I realized what a valuable historical record it is. The messages (and the journal entries), written in the midst of the battle, convey the experience, day-by-day, even hour-by-hour at times, with remarkable immediacy. It is as close to being there as is possible, I believe. I hope that for those of you who read it, the book will provide information, knowledge, insight, and strength that will help you in your struggle against a hidden, deadly foe that even today confounds the best minds in medical science and research. And I especially hope that even though Stella and I lost our battle, our story may still inspire others to fight with all their hearts and souls to overcome the negativity they so often face and to escape the death sentence they've been given. No one—not even the most renowned physician—can say with certainty who may succeed against all the odds.

◆   ◆   ◆

Knowing how little time patients and caregivers have to read anything, I wanted to make it as easy as possible to find subjects that may be of immediate interest. For that reason, I've done a fairly extensive index. Also, I divided the book into three sections, which are set out in the Table of Contents and which I hope will help guide readers in finding quickly the information they seek.

Section 1. The First Nine Months

Fri Mar 26 1999 2:01 PM

Peggy—I'm sorry I haven't been in today. I came to the Gallery yesterday but went home still not feeling all that great. I'm still battling what appears to be a sinus infection. I've been thinking that it would be helpful for me at some point to have a better sense of how you go about planning a regular screening program. I'm wondering if it would be possible to sit in on a couple of meetings that you may be having as you put together a schedule. I'd like to get a sense of what the problems and steps are. If there should be an opportunity for this, let me know. Many thanks, Stel

NOTE: Stel was planning a film program for the National Gallery of Art, which is what the above message relates to. The "sinus infection" she thought was causing her problems was actually referred pain from the tumor in her right frontal lobe, as we found out a month later. During this same period, she was putting together a five-hour presentation on documentary film for a graduate history class at American University. That is the subject of the messages immediately following.

Tue Apr 20 1999 11:11 PM

Dear Stel, I want to thank you again for your superb presentation tonight. It was a real pleasure and a learning experience from which we all benefitted tremendously. It is clear that you worked far too hard, but it paid off. See you tomorrow. Best, Vanessa

Wed Apr 21 1999 9:36 AM

Dear Vanessa, I appreciated your response and that of the class. It was an experience for me on a subject I've been dying to get into and you gave me that opportunity. I couldn't sleep thinking of all the points I wished I had made, but another time. Thanks again, Stel

NOTE: Stel forwarded the message from Vanessa to me at work and the message below was my response. Stel never saw it because she had already left for lunch and had no chance to look at e-mail when she returned home feeling ill.

Wed Apr 21 1999 12:36 PM

I'm so delighted, Stella, that for once you're getting the recognition you deserve. Coming from Vanessa, who, I'm sure, is a tough critic of such presentations, it means a lot. Love, Kay

NOTE: After the ER visit on April 21st and her MRI on the 22nd, Stel and I saw the neurosurgeon recommended by her internist, Dr. Arthur Kobrine, on April 26th. He told Stel the tumor wasn't life threatening yet but it would be soon. By the time she left his office that day, she had scheduled surgery for ten days later.

Wed Apr 28 1999 10:40 AM

Dear Cathy, Just have a minute. I've wanted to call you. Regarding summer plans, I've just learned that I must have surgery. It's scheduled for May 6. I can't make plans and feel very bad about not being able to tell you anything at this time. But it appears as though I may not be able to make the trip. Hope to talk to you more via phone. Love to family, Stel

Thu Apr 29 1999 6:42 AM

Dear Peggy, First, I've done some editing of the film notes you gave me and will turn in the draft later today. Second, quite unexpectedly and to my great distress, I just learned that I will have to have some surgery next week and have been very busy with preparations for this. I'm very upset at the break this will mean for the Cacoyannis project I've been involved with since I won't be up and fully functioning for several weeks. Assuming things proceed as I expect they will, I would hope to be able to continue working on the various details involved with that program in a few weeks. Even if at home, I could draft the necessary program notes. Since I suggested the program, I feel responsible for it and would hope to be able to carry through after this hiatus.

Finally, regarding the city films program idea with Vanessa, I will let her know my situation today or tomorrow. I'm sure that she would have no problem writing something up in a couple of pages with her suggestions for films and a unifying theme. Of course, I would love to work with her on any future film and lecture programming as we had discussed at lunch and will hope to do so as soon as I am able. I really regret having to suspend my work with you for the moment. I've enjoyed it and hope I've been of some help.—Stel

Thu Apr 29 1999 5:39 PM

Dear Stel: I want you to know that I will do anything I can to help you through this very difficult time. You are an incredibly strong individual to have given no indication of what was going on at lunch last Wednesday. You gave such a great presentation Tuesday night. I was just amazed that you had the energy to come to the Gallery the next morning. I can't imagine all the work you put into that five-hour lecture, and it was as smooth as silk. I took the most notes I have ever taken in that class! And then to have symptoms the next day. You gave no indication of what you were going through. You should get the Academy Award! Please let me do whatever I can for you. I really value our friendship and want to be there at the hospital when you have surgery and want to help out afterward when you are recuperating. Love, Linda.

Thu Apr 29 1999 7:31 PM

Dear Linda, What can I say? Kay and I deeply appreciate your caring spirit. It would mean so much to Kay (and of course to me) for you to be there, if you can. But I am concerned about your work and your paper, so be wise with your time, please. Our friend Chris Carroll, the artist, will be coming for a couple of days and this is a strange way for you to meet, but who can predict life? I spoke briefly to Peggy today. I just want you to know, as I told her, that I've valued this experience and the chance to be there. I worked hard but I wish I could have accomplished more. I am deeply upset at having to leave some things hanging, but hope to pick up where I left off, and if your good spiritual vibes carry any weight, I shall. Thank you for your friendship—from both of us, Stel

Sun May 02 1999 11:33 PM

Dear Renata, I'm sorry to report some bad news. I've had to cancel my trip because Stel has been diagnosed with a brain tumor and is going to have surgery on May 6th. Needless to say, this is all very unexpected and upsetting. It's impossible to know at this point whether the tumor is cancerous or not. Stel has always been very healthy and all of her other tests are showing things as normal, so I believe in my heart that she will come through okay. But we won't know for sure what the situation is until after the surgery, which will take about five hours. Stel is being incredibly brave about it, but I just feel so bad that she has to go through this awful procedure. She's never even been in the hospital before. I'm taking the whole month of May off to stay home during her recuperation, and will take longer if necessary. Fortunately, we have some good friends who have been wonderful support and will be with me at the hospital while the operation is going on. Stel's cousin will also be here from Michigan.

This is all like a very bad dream and I keep thinking we'll wake up from it and I'll find myself happily planning for my trip. Unfortunately, there's no waking up. The fact of it just keeps staring us in the face. I only wish I'd be seeing you as we planned. Hopefully, both Stel and I can get to Germany within the year. Nothing would make me happier at this point than to be able to plan a trip with her soon. I guess that's all I can say for now. I'll let you know as soon as I know what the results of the surgery are. As I say, I expect things to turn out all right in the end. Stel sends you her best. Love, Kay

Mon May 03 1999 11:44 PM

Dear Edie, This all began about two weeks ago. We saw the neurosurgeon a week ago today. He said there's a very remote possibility that it's an infection, but he doesn't think so because she's not in any of the risk groups for that. More likely, according to the MRI technician, is either a glioma or a meningioma. It's about golf-ball size, deep, but fortunately on her non-dominant side and in the frontal lobe in front of the motor apparatus. The surgeon, who is one of the best in the country according to people we've talked to, thinks he can get to it without hurting her much—there's a 5% chance of some weakness on the left side. We talked about doing a biopsy, but it doesn't seem to offer much advantage and has the disadvantage of having her go through two awful hospital procedures. She's doing okay—no more dizzy spells or numbness, some twinges on her left side. And she's very tired, not all of which is attributable to this, I think. She's had an exhausting several months. She's being quite brave about it, but, of course is scared, as am I. I don't believe in my heart that it will turn out to be a really bad tumor. Stel is in good shape, as all the doctors have noted, and I don't think is prone to malignant growths.

She's going to get a second opinion tomorrow, but I think it's likely she'll go through with surgery on May 6th. We feel pretty confident in the neurosurgeon, whom we've seen twice, and in the hospital—Georgetown. Also some of the stuff we've read about tumors and the treatment of them indicates that surgery is probably what should be done. Fortunately, our friend Chris from Berkeley will be here during surgery, as will her cousin. And a couple of other good friends from here. Needless to say, this last ten days has been a nightmare, and I keep thinking we'll wake up from it, but no such luck. I'll let you know how the surgery goes on Thursday. Love, Kay

Wed May 05, 1999 3:57 PM

Dear Deborah, I'm violating Stel's wishes to let you know that in the last two weeks she was diagnosed with a brain tumor and is being operated on tomorrow morning at Georgetown Hospital. We won't know until after the operation—and for perhaps up to a week—what the nature of the tumor is, but we're hoping for the best. And I believe it will be the best, or close to it. She's a healthy person and I can't believe she has been invaded by an aggressively malignant growth. She's been remarkably strong about it. She has a top-notch doctor and hospital and therefore is in the best hands she can be in.

I'm sorry to send this bad news, but I thought you'd want to know. I'll let you know as soon as we know what the results are. Since we don't seem to be waking up from this nightmare, we'll try to do the next best thing and deal with what has to be dealt with as positively as we can. All the best, Kay

Thu May 06 1999 1:53 AM

Martha, Surgery is at 7:30 AM—probably lasting until 12:30 or so. Please channel those good wishes—and I'll tell Stel to visualize a teddy bear holding her in a big bear hug the whole time. She's brave, and with all the positive energy coming from so many people, plus her own fighting spirit, I think she'll come through okay. More later, Kay

Thu May 06 1999 11:32 PM

Dear Martha, The good news is Stel came through the operation very well. She got an A+ from the doctor. Only an hour or so after the operation, she was lucid and loquacious, and rather stoned, as we talked in the IC unit. She said she deserved a medal, and we agree and are going to try to find one for her. She was very relieved it was over.

The less good news is that the initial pathology report indicated that the tumor was not benign. It may be a #3 or 4 malignancy, which is bad, but we won't know for sure for a week. I'm praying it may be a #2 and at most a #3. Whatever it is, it means follow-up radiation and maybe other things. Stel doesn't know this and I hope she doesn't push for an answer from me for a couple of days anyway. I'm heartbroken that she has to go through more shit. I really had believed it would be benign; at least I thought the odds were against anything really bad because she already had so many losses in her family—her youngest brother, two nieces and a nephew (the latest niece last week), and others in the past 15 or so years. But the deck has always seemed to be stacked against her.

We had wonderful support from friends and family today and are grateful for that. At this point, I can't envision what the future holds for us, my work, etc. I guess the next few weeks will tell. Love, Kay

Mon May 10 1999 2:17 PM

Dear Ruth, Thanks so much for your note. It's amazing how many stories we've heard since Stel was diagnosed about people of all ages and in all stages of brain tumors who have survived and thrived. We certainly intend for Stel to be among them. Fortunately, she came through the surgery like a champ; all the doctors and nurses in the hospital were telling her how brave she was and how strong her body was. And they were equally impressed with her progress in recovering from the operation. She was in good enough shape to be released from the hospital yesterday and, needless to say, we're both glad she's home in her own bedroom. I had hoped so much that the tumor would be benign, but apparently it isn't. We'll find out on Friday what we're facing, although the surgeon seemed to be signalling that it's either going to be bad or very bad. But whatever it is, we'll fight it. And we've had such an outpouring of love and support from so many friends and acquaintances, which makes a very terrifying time a little easier to bear. I'll give Stel your good wishes and appreciate your offer of help. Love, Kay

Mon May 10 1999 7:29 PM

Vanessa, We've found out that Stel's appointment with her doctor will be on Friday morning, when we'll probably get the results of the final path report. I just sent a message to Deborah about whether she will be available that day if Stel feels she would like to talk to her after that dreaded session. I'm sending this message to ask you the same question, I believe very strongly that your friendship and support for Stel during this horrible time can make a significant difference, whatever we learn on Friday—and I'm hoping beyond hope that we'll have the best news we can get at this point—that the grade of tumor she has is manageable for some years to come. My deepest thanks, Kay

Wed May 12 1999 3:45 PM

Dear Vanessa, Thanks so much for the offer of food. I think we're fixed fine for the moment since Stel's cousin is still here. He is an excellent cook, a blessing for us all, but especially Stel, given the less than excellent quality of my culinary skills. She's doing phenomenally well—even insisted on getting down on the floor a few minutes ago to fix the answering machine—which she did after I had made a vain effort. We took a short walk outside today as well. She's now taking a rest after all her exertions but wanted me to send you this note (which she scribbled out) from her: Dear Prof. Vanessa, Your visit at the hospital with Deborah lifted my spirits and the vision of your two smiling faces is still with me. I think you know how much your friendship means to me. I feel so lucky to have had a chance to share so many ideas with you about film, history, life. Your devoted student, Stel

Wed May 12 1999 5:36 PM

Dear Linda, I'm already benefiting from your many gifts—the tea (digestion much better), lip balm (lips now nearly healed), Dr. Weil's great healing book which Kay and I are both devouring. I can't believe how much you pulled out of your huge cache of gifts Monday night. You've brought us so much happiness and so many good times with you. Your incredible generosity, kindness, and caring are great boons to us and we're grateful to have your friendship. I hope I have a chance to give back just a little of the generosity you've showered on me. With love, Stel

Thu May 13 1999 6:38 PM

Dear Stel, I'm so glad you're back at the keyboard! We had a small gathering at Vanessa's house last night for the last class. I talked with Vanessa about the film program and took notes furiously. I think I understood what she was proposing. But would you mind if I sent you a draft of this proposal and you could finalize it with her? If you're not up to it then I'll just slog along. But I really don't know anything about city films, the history of film or anything. Let me know if you mind reviewing e-mails to get this started. Love, Linda

Thu May 13 1999 9:48 PM

Dear Deborah, Stel is recovering very nicely. She's up wandering around the apartment by herself today, and yesterday we took a short walk outside. Also, her spirits are high. She's had wonderful messages from a host of friends, and our place is inundated with flowers and plants. She and I have also been reading a book Linda gave us by Dr. Andrew Weil on <u>Spontaneous Healing</u> which lays out specific ways to strengthen your immune system and body and we've already embarked on some of his suggestions. We're determined that whatever we hear tomorrow, we're going to come out in a fighting spirit and do everything we can to ensure that Stel beats the odds. Of course, in the middle of the night when we both wake up to demons, it's not so easy to keep that resolve. But we just get up and talk, remember all the wonderful places we've been together, talk about the Dodd project, watch TV, and finally get tired enough to sleep again.

Anyway, please just keep thinking "No more than #3" tomorrow morning and maybe all our thinking will make it so. If so, the road ahead will look a bit less scary. Stel and I both look forward to seeing you and Vanessa and Linda tomorrow. With love and thanks, Kay

Thu May 13 1999 9:58 PM

Dear Linda, We'll be in touch with you after the doctor's appointment. Stel's spirits are good, as are mine, and we're determined to come out fighting no matter what we hear. But to have you and Vanessa and Deborah around later in the day will be a great boost. (Just keep thinking "no more than #3" tomorrow morning and maybe all our vibes will make it so.)

Stel wanted me to tell you that she'd love to look at the draft of the proposal (and I think it would be great for her to have that to concentrate on). Also, she and I were bowled over by the gorgeous floral arrangement that arrived today. She has many beautiful flowers and plants, but that outstrips them all. Love, Kay

<u>NOTE</u>: We saw Stel's neurosurgeon on May 14th and he told us that the final pathology report indicated the tumor was grade IV, a glioblastoma multiforme. However, he said he had "held the tumor in his hand" and it "didn't look as ugly" as the worst ones usually do—it was a grey, gelatinous mass rather than a yellowish, greenish, blackish one. Stel and I were very encouraged by that because we felt he didn't really believe the path report. We asked him to get a second opinion. He also referred her to an oncologist he often worked with, saying they had had great success in treating other GBM patients and would work as a team to do everything they could for her.

Sun May 16 1999 6:14 PM

Dear Vanessa, I hope next Thursday night at six is okay with you—at your place. Kay and I are looking forward to getting out and having such great company. A real salon event. Linda can join us from 6-8 PM, and I may not last any longer. Also, I know you must be busy preparing for your trip, but is there any way we can talk, even on the phone about the memo to Peggy re city films and your lecture(s). Linda sent me her notes after meeting with you and I have time now to draft something simple, but will need further discussion with you. Love, Stel

Mon May 17 1999 5:32 PM

Dear Madeleine and Jerry, Thanks so much for your kind message. It's wonderful to hear from you. As Peter told you, I am doing well after the surgery. My spirits are high because I have so many wonderful friends who have called, sent messages, come by—all encouraging me to get well and stimulating me with ideas and interesting projects. I know that encouragement, along with my excellent doctors, will help me do what I have to do to recover fully. Kay and I are looking forward eagerly to returning to beautiful Stockholm to visit good friends like you. I long to be there. I'll keep you posted on my progress and when I'm booking my flight to Sweden. Love, Stel

Tue May 18 1999 2:40 PM

Dear Stel, Thank you for your wonderful, wonderful mail! We were so happy to hear from you so quickly. You sound so full of fighting spirit, just like we knew you would. You are strong Stel and it must be great to have a person like Kay by your side right now. Let's keep in touch. Lots of love to you and Kay, Madeleine and Jerry

Sat May 22 1999 12:38 PM

Dear Vanessa, The Peggy memo is great. I think she will really be pleased. You added just the right things. I'll e-mail her and let you know what she says. I'm so excited to think we may have a program here. It really makes me happy. This is an opportunity too to tell you again how much I enjoyed the Thursday gathering. I've been around many Hollywood types, but the company at your table was more stellar. I appreciate, as you know, your support and love and friendship. Have a great trip and I look forward to your postcards from Paris. Stella

Sat May 22 1999 12:52 PM

Dear Stig, I was so happy to hear from you and appreciate your kind concern about my present state. Actually, I feel great. The operation went extremely well and though I will have to undergo treatments (radiation, and perhaps some chemotherapy), my body and spirit are good and I intend to keep feeling this way. My only problem is that I am in the wrong country! I'd love to be in Sweden, my favorite place. I'd feel a lot better to be away from American violence, guns and killing. When I begin to fantazise, I always think of beautiful Stockholm and the many great people there. A visit to Stockholm is definitely in my future and I look forward to spending time with my friends there. With love and kisses, Stel

NOTE: On May 19—thirteen days after Stel's surgery and five days after her surgeon had delivered the bad news of the final path report—the doctor called her to give her more "bad news." Listening in on the other phone, I heard him tell her that all of the tumor except the tiny frozen section had been lost by the nurse who was supposed to take it to the lab from the operating room. Our impression was that he had just learned about this. In fact, as we later found out, he had known about it since the afternoon of the surgery on May 6th. At the time, we thought it was an odd thing to happen but accepted his explanation without question.

Mon May 24 1999 9:04 PM

Dear Edie, Sorry not to have gotten back to you sooner. The days fly by, even though they're no fun, and I find myself collapsing into bed every night without having accomplished half of what I thought I would that day. The news has been mixed, and we've got a difficult road ahead. The final path report came back with the worst—a four—but Stel's surgeon said, from his years of experience and thousands of tumors he's seen, that it didn't look as "ugly" as the worst tumors usually look. We took a lot of hope in that. We're going to have a second path report done, but we're girding ourselves for it to come back the same. They'll be testing the same small sample again. If you can believe it, the hospital lost the rest of the tumor the surgeon removed—somewhere between the operating room and the lab. The surgeon was so furious he got a nurse fired over it. At any rate, that means there's nothing else to test; it also means the surgeon is the only one who saw this not so "ugly" tumor.

If it really is a four, Stel is in for a fight for her life because they tend to grow back rapidly, despite treatment. However, her surgeon and the oncologist he sent her to have a very good track record with extending the lives of many people with these tumors by several years [according to him]. If it's a three, the odds improve significantly with treatment. The treatment is the same for both—radiation and chemo. She starts radiation next Thursday. It's five days a week for six to seven weeks. After that, the oncologist will decide about chemo. There is the outside chance that he might look at the MRI after the radiation and decide there's no need for chemo, but more than likely he'll want her to have three rounds of about a month apiece. She's upset about that prospect and so am I, but we'll cross that bridge when we come to it.

The other good news we got from the oncologist and the radiation oncologist is that the tumor was on the small side and there's a direct correlation between size and survival rates.[1] Also the radiation oncologist confirmed the surgeon's view by saying that the tumor didn't look like the worst type on the MRI itself. So we hold to these slender threads and are doing a pretty good job so far of keeping our spirits up—with the help of a lot of friends. I'm also filling her full of as many good things—organic fruits, veggies, herbs, vitamins, etc.—as I can think of.

I have no idea how I'm going to work a forty-hour week at the same time, but I've got to try. I'm taking two more weeks of leave, which I still have, for the first two weeks of June. Then I've proposed to my boss spending twelve hours a week in the office and telecommuting the rest. She's considering this and I guess I'll hear further in a few days. If this doesn't work, though, I'm just going to have to take a leave without pay, which is not going to do our already battered finances any good. But first things first, and Stel's first by a long shot. Love, Kay

Wed May 26 1999 5:19 AM

Dear George [Stel's cousin], It was great, as usual, to talk to you. I always learn so much from our talks. However, I do apologize if I distressed you with my tears. Actually, I'm in a surprisingly good mood, considering my situation and I believe this is partly a result of the strong support I've had from so many friends—even as far away as Stockholm! In all the literature I've read, this is key. There's no way to thank you for your kindness and support all these years. But I do have a little gift which I hope you'll enjoy—designed by my dear friend in California. (It's a "music muffler," which patrons of the arts and musicians are crazy about.) It's not wrapped. I really tried and had beautiful paper, but alas, it would not fit into

---

1. This is what the oncologist said explicitly to Stel and the radiation oncologist seemed to concur. I never saw any research that made such a finding, and no other doctor ever told us this.

my envelope. So you'll just have to imagine that it comes with much love. I hope it reaches you before you leave for Greece. I'd love to be in Crete. Perhaps this is in my future. I want so much to finish my Greek language studies and this will be a spur to get well. Love and kalo taxidi, Stella

Sat May 29 1999 10:35 PM

Dear George, I forgot to enclose the beautiful card I had to go along with the "music muffler." Don't forget to let me know your date of departure. Feeling good and hope you are too. I have so much to do. The film curator at the National Gallery of Art liked my proposal for another program that brings together Paris in the 20s, films about Paris and several lectures by one of my professors who is a talented speaker. This makes me very happy. Fortunately, this part of my brain is still percolating with ideas! Love, Stella

NOTE: Stel and I refer in several messages below to a trip we took over Memorial Day weekend, at the invitation of our friend Linda, to a cabin in the West Virginia mountains. Stel's friend, Cathy, was visiting for those days and came with us. A few days before the trip, Stel had been running a temperature and a doctor had thought she might have an infection. We were relieved when the fever went away in a couple of days, but then the day we planned to drive to West Virginia, Stel woke up with a rash on her face and body. After urgent calls to the doctor on duty over that holiday weekend, it was determined that she was having a reaction to her seizure medication, Dilantin, and she was switched to Tegretol. The doctor recommended to her that she not go on the trip, but she decided to go anyway and it was a great respite for us.

Wed Jun 02 1999 7:05 PM

Dear Linda, The three of us want to thank you profusely for the wonderful weekend you provided. For me, I think it was so therapeutic and the point at which I really have felt a definite breakthrough. My fever is gone and so nearly is my rash. I'm so glad I followed my instinct that the clean air, the great company and the change of pace—and just escaping dire phone calls from doctors—would improve my attitude. And the experience did just that. The condo was comfy, and Richard's cuisine kept us all healthy and pampered. Kay, too, benefited from the therapeutic weekend and got some much needed rest, not to mention the pleasure of your company. Cathy was equally thrilled to meet you and Richard and had a wonderful time. It was a lot of fun! And we did have a lot of laughs. Love, Stel and Kay

Thu Jun 03 1999 7:15 AM

Dear Linda, As Stel has already told you in her e-mail, the trip was a real tonic, and respite, for us. We really got to relax, feel "normal," and forget almost entirely about our worries. We came back feeling rested and strong. And we, too, had a very good time with you and Richard—good company, interesting conversation, and yummy food is a combination that can't be beat. Thanks so-o-o-o much. Stel begins radiation this morning at 11 AM. Until later, Kay

Fri Jun 04 1999 6:15 PM

Dear Cathy, It's not the same here without you. You were great and helped me feel so much stronger. I was thinking about our weekend and how perfectly you joined in with us. I can't thank you enough for caring about me and my illness. When I got back I felt that I had made a real breakthrough. I'm feeling more and more like my old self—so much so that I don't or can't believe I have what they say I have. I've had two sessions of radiation thus far and so we shall see in a couple of weeks just what impact this is having on those awful cells. My good feeling and spirit must have some relationship to the condition of my brain, but I don't want to be too cocky until I see how I fare with the chemotherapy, in the event they do that to me. Enough about me. I hope your flight back was good. All my love, Stella

Sat Jun 05 1999 8:54 AM

Dear Madeleine and Jerry, It's so much fun to hear news from friends abroad. I hope you have a great time in Portugal. This past weekend a good friend rented a condo in West Virginia—about 4 hours away—and invited us. I came back feeling so much better. Now I'm really beginning to get my strength back—so much so that I sometimes forget that I was even in the hospital. Perhaps I'm not facing reality. I don't know, but my surgeon believes I must continue to maintain a positive attitude and I like him a lot. There is something to this mind over matter business. So while I'm feeling good, I want to write as much as I can. Lots of love from Kay and me, Stella

Tue Jun 08 1999 2:35 PM

Dear Cathy, Thanks so much for your good message. As usual, I'm doing too many things in too many directions. Like yesterday, I was calling Athens and Paris to reach Cacoyannis, who I finally did talk to. There's plenty more detail to handle on this particular program. Many thanks for your caring efforts in helping me. I realize more and more how important my friends have been in stimulating my enthusiasm for life. Love from Stel (and Kay)

Wed Jun 09 1999 6:38 PM

Dear Vanessa, What a great pleasure to hear from you. Yes, we received your gorgeous postcard. I wanted to tell you that Peggy loved our "city films" memo and it looks like the program is a go. On other fronts: I've also been able to pick up where I left off on the Cacoyannis program. I've been a busy girl, so much so, that I sometimes forget that I've had major surgery and am now in radiation. I'm up and about and I really believe it's due in large part to great, wonderful friends like you. Your attention and concern and encouragement (and Kay's constant care) have been the best medicine and stimulus I could have hoped for.

I'm nearing the end of my first week of radiation. I begin the morning at Georgetown as Frankenstein (they place a marked and colored mask over my face & strap me in to keep the beams precise). After a few zaps, really only a couple of minutes, I'm released. I feel a little lightheaded afterwards, but nothing more difficult than that. I hope it all continues to be as easily tolerated as this first period.

Let me know if we can be of any help on this end. I've collected a couple of articles that may interest you and will save them for your return. Lots of love & hugs from us both, Stel and Kay

Mon Jun 14 1999 2:21 PM

Dear Cathy, I'm sending you much love and thanks for all your help. I love that you're sending me loving thoughts. I can use all I can get. I have finished my first big week of radiation and my doctor (very young and not so traditional) has cut down my steroid medication so I'm only taking half of what I was on. I was thrilled and hope I don't slip back. I'm sorry it took me so long to write. You would have to be here to understand why. My therapy, the phones, the friends, the food, the caring that one single person needs. How do people manage without the support I've received? Love, Stella

Wed Jun 16 1999 8:30 AM

Dear Moira, Glad to hear from you. I'm just realizing that my left hand doesn't work as well as the right on the computer so it slows me down. It will pass with more working out. I've been doing pretty good. Yesterday was terrible, however, but I suspect it was because my doctor was trying to wean me off the steroids and dropped my medication just enough to make it quite difficult for me. So I'll have to wait a bit. But she is very wise and good to do this and understands the problems with steroids so I admire her effort. I got a good rest last night and today feel much better. I will call you this weekend. Keep up the good work! If Elaine can pass her qualifying orals for the Ph.D, so can Moira. Love, Stel

Wed Jun 16 1999 8:41 AM

Dear Rosemary, Yes, last week was very good for me. This week, with the accumulation of the radiation and the way it reddens your scalp was a bit more difficult. Yesterday I did not sleep and they increased my medication which they had decreased the day before. So last night I slept well and feel good this morning. Thanks for all your caring and concern. I'm collecting all these good thoughts. Love from me, too, Stella

Thu Jun 17 1999 5:22 PM

Dear Cathy, I've completed my second week of radiation and it's very time-consuming and tiring. I'll give you a call over the weekend. I know you're getting excited about your trip. I'm so glad you'll stay in touch with me. That really helps a lot, and I'll be anxious to hear the details of the house and village you're in and who you meet and so forth. So I'm looking forward to this almost as much as you, vicariously. Lots of love from me and Kay, Stella

Thu Jun 24 1999 8:00 AM

Dear Deborah, A short note to say you were wise not to attend the lecture last night. I'm sad to report that it was disappointing. He didn't seem to have a strong thesis. I have to tell you your strawberries were fantastic and in the middle of the night, a chunk of the calamata bread soothed the hole in my stomach and got me back to sleep. But your visit was most beneficent. Love, Stella

Thu Jun 24 1999 1:46 PM

Dear Kat, Regarding last night, I saw you below us [at the lecture at the U.S. Holocaust Museum]. We got there very late after wrestling with terrible traffic. I was frankly disappointed with the lecture and will be very interested to hear your response to it. I had looked forward to the reception afterwards but was so tired and not feeling so great that we decided to take off. So I'm sorry to have missed you. Let me know when you can either come over for dinner or meet us for lunch or dinner at that place in Dupont Circle, whichever you prefer. Best regards, Stel

<u>NOTE</u>: Stel refers in the message below to seeing her oncologist. This was midway through radiation treatment. He told us that the second path report on the tiny tumor sample also found a grade IV tumor, but emphasized that it was small and circumscribed, which boded well for treatment. "The less cancer you're dealing with the better." He checked Stel out physically and found improvement in her symptoms that was "extremely encouraging." Things were "going extremely well," he said. I asked him what that meant and he responded that it could mean either the swelling and/or the tumor cells were receding, or that the cells were "starting to resume normal function." At a minimum, he said, it told him that "the tumor isn't growing and not getting worse." It showed a good response to radiation, which was "very encouraging." He talked, as he had at Stel's first appointment, of PCV treatment after radiation but said, in response to a question from Stel, that he wouldn't start chemo if the MRI about a month after radiation showed dramatic improvement. Despite the bad news about the second path report, we left the session feeling buoyed and very hopeful.

Tue Jun 29 1999 7:30 AM

Dear George, Thanks so much for your help with the property. I hope you're having a great time in Crete. Wish I were there. I saw my oncologist yesterday and he was very, very pleased with my progress. Coming from this very reserved scientist (who I call Dr. Freud because he looks like him), it made me feel great. So all steam ahead! Love from this side of the Atlantic, Stella

Tue Jun 29 1999 7:56 PM

Dear Madeleine, Thank you so much for your wonderful messages and for looking for the translation for me. I look forward to reading the play. I saw my doctor yesterday, and he was very encouraged at how well I am doing half way through the radiation treatment. It will be finished in three weeks and we'll see what the next steps are. One of my most pleasant thoughts these days is of Stockholm and visiting with my friends there. Kay and I look forward to making those daydreams a reality. Kay sends her love, as do I. Stella

Fri Jul 02 1999 10:01 PM

Dear Deborah, Regarding our plans for the 4th [July 4th was Stel's birthday], it seems the forecast thus far is for 99 degree weather. So I doubt that we should consider barbequeing in such heat and humidity, much as I would like to. We'll just buy some rotisserie chickens and I'll make a big salad, as we discussed. But we can talk about this when you get back. Warmest regards from Kay & me, Stel

Mon Jul 05 1999 6:41 PM

Dear Cathy, It sounds as though you've already had great experiences. Your images have given me a lot to visualize. Thank you. As for radiation, I've completed more than half of the therapy. It does tire me and I feel so much time wasted in running back and forth to the hospital. I'm having a little trouble with my left side, getting my left hand fingers to work better on the computer keyboard. However, if I keep at my exercises, this all seems to diminish. I'm so impatient to return my body completely to normal.

Chris was here for my birthday and last night Deborah graciously opened her home to about nine of us to gather for the 4th. It was exceedingly hot and everyone's energy was flagging. I wanted to make a little speech but didn't and felt bad about it. But this is just the kind of thing I have to avoid feeling. The self-criticism. It does no good. Love to you all, Stella

Mon Jul 05 1999 9:56 PM

Dear George, I won't write much except to say I only have about eight more radiation treatments to go. It's really been a drain, Monday through Friday every week for the past five, but now it's thankfully downhill and we shall see what lies ahead. I'm a little fatigued but I must continue with my good diet (no sugar, a difficult thing for me). Lots of veggies and fruits, but no desserts. My oncologist says if my MRI is really good he will reconsider chemotherapy. I'm working hard to make this happen. Since I have a few weeks before chemo would begin, I'm going to fortify my body with all the good supplements I haven't been able to have because the doctors felt it might interfere with the radiation.[2] Love, Stella

Wed Jul 07 1999 12:34 PM

Dear Linda, I hope you're feeling much better now. I just returned from a treatment and am a bit spacey but wanted to thank you (again and again) for your lovely little gifts of soaps and salts. They're wonderful in the bath. As to our gathering at Deborah's house on the 4th, I'm afraid I just wasn't up to much joyful

---

2. The radiation oncologist had told Stel not to take large doses of vitamin C or E because of concern as to how anti-oxidants might adversely affect the radiation. So far as I know, there is no conclusive scientific evidence of such an effect.

conversation. I had so looked forward to this gathering, but by the time it happened, I was more fatigued than I wished to admit. I had even drafted a little speech in my head about how I was surrounded by such great people who had all returned from wonderful trips—but just couldn't bring myself to recite it. I hope Kay and I will have a chance to hear more details of your adventures and the people you met. Perhaps when you get some rest. Love, Stel

Tue Jul 13 1999 9:47 PM

Dear Madeleine, Thanks so much for the opportunity to read the play. I really enjoyed the characters and admired Gertrude for having the courage to walk away from her husband, despite her misfired romance. The play gave me some insight into the Swedish male-female mentality and it sounds very familiar on this side of the Atlantic.

I just wanted to mention that I have nearly completed my radiation treatments and will have done so by July 21. Then I have several weeks break while the doctors determine how next to proceed. So far, they are telling me I'm doing great and this gives me hope. I don't like the idea of having to do chemotherapy, but this treatment in combination with the radiation appears to have a success record with patients who have conditions similar to mine. So I will try to prepare myself for this next phase. Thank you so much for mentioning the anecdote of your friend who had breast cancer and is surviving. This is very inspiring to me. Lots of love and appreciation, Stel (and Kay)

Tue July 20 1999 4:02 PM

Dear Vanessa, How kind of you to call and check up on me. Only two more days of radiation treatments. So far all is going well. I'm tired but that's a small price to pay, I feel. We're meeting at Linda's tomorrow evening for a potluck (to celebrate the end of radiation). Wish you could be with us. I hope you're getting some rest and sleep while you can. Lots of love and good wishes from me and Kay, Stel

Sat Jul 24 1999 3:23 PM

Dear Kat, What a pleasure to hear from you! And to learn of your adventures. We had a dinner with some friends the other evening and you were sorely missed. But we look forward to seeing you on your return. I've now completed my radiation phase of therapy, over these past seven weeks and am very relieved. They are giving me a break of about a month. I plan to try to get over the radiation and pull myself together in this time, eat all the vitamins I can possibly consume and get ready for what is next. All you're missing here is hot and humid weather which doesn't quit. Love from Kay & me, Stel

Sat July 24 1999 3:34 PM

Dear Cathy, I owe you such a long letter after the wonderful ones you've sent me. We've had guests. Kay's sister came after Chris and you and began to teach me some piano for my keyboard. I want you to know that I have now concluded my radiation therapy! And I will have a break of some four weeks or so. Kay is feeding me potent stuff, the best vitamins (selenium plus E, and great teas). I've got my foot propped up and when I feel more rested I'll write again. Just wanted you to know you're in my thoughts and that I love you, Stella

Thu July 29 1999 9:16 AM

Dear Cathy, You've been great about keeping me informed and I have been very bad on my end. Some of this has to do with my time. Healing oneself takes all day long! And I have Kay to help me. She is a godsend. She's done so much research for me and has found through Lerner's great book an outpatient operation run by Dr. Keith Block in Illinois.[3] It sounds right for me and we're scheduled to be there on the 19th of August. Will report back on this experience. A second problem apart from limited time to write to you is that I continue to have a slowness in my left hand and fingers, so when I'm on the computer keyboard, it all becomes laborious to type and I'm less inclined to do so. I know your stay is drawing to a close, and wish it were longer. I'll call you on your return. If you receive this, know that I've been thinking about all of you and wish you a safe return home—and a return to Europe maybe next year? Love and good wishes, Stella

Sun Aug 01 1999 3:52 PM

Dear Kat, We're doing fine here. I finished radiation ten days ago and am so glad not to be going to those sessions every morning. I'm taking all my vitamins, minerals, herbs, enzymes, etc., as directed. I have no choice with my food policeman Kay around all the time. I'm feeling well, although tired, and am going to an acupunturist and Chinese herbal doctor to find out what he can do for me. On

---

3.   Block Center for Integrative Cancer Care, Evanston, Illinois; 847-492-3040; www.blockmd.com

August 19th Kay and I will go to Chicago for an appointment with a doctor there who has a very holistic approach to dealing with cancer and I think I'll learn a lot from that. By the end of August I'll know whether my oncologist is going to recommend chemotherapy and I want to be armed with as much information as I can before then. Stay in touch. Warm wishes, Stel

Wed Aug 04 1999 3:47 PM

Dear Deborah, Thanks so much for a delightful afternoon. It was so much fun to be with you. I had a thought regarding film: I'd like you to see Kevin Brownlow's Cinema Europe series—at least the part on Germany and France. I believe there's interesting footage there that pertains to the inter-war period. You should be familiar with the Brownlow series. He's a wonderful preservationist, writer and filmmaker. If you get this in time, send me again the name of the film on men you want me to check. This is a good excuse to visit the Motion Picture Reading Room/LOC to talk to the staff and check their catalogues. Have good trips. Love, Stel

NOTE: About 10:30 PM on the evening of August 6th, Stel had a focal seizure on her left side (her first). We put in an emergency call to her neurosurgeon, who rudely told Stel (I was on the other phone) that he hadn't "seen [her] in months and didn't have any idea what was happening." He told her she should go to an emergency room. Shocked at his coldness, I called 911 and rushed her to the ER where we had gone on the night of April 21st. A CT scan showed extensive swelling of the brain. The ER doctor telephoned Dr. Kobrine in the early hours of the morning to tell him that his patient should be admitted to the hospital for observation. He assumed that the doctor would want to have Stel transferred to Georgetown Hospital—20 minutes away—where the surgery had been done in May. Dr. Kobrine refused to take her in transfer. When the ER doctor, incredulous, asked whether Dr. Kobrine agreed that the patient required acute hospitalization, according to his ER report, Dr. Kobrine said, "Yes she does, by your neurosurgeon. I am telling you I will not accept her in transfer." (I was standing beside the ER doctor as he had this very brief conversation. He was livid when he got off the phone.) The doctor told us the substance of the conversation and recommended that Stel get another neurosurgeon. We immediately opted for Dr. Melissa Neiman, whom Stel had consulted for a second opinion and who worked out of the local hospital. The next day, after she had reviewed the MRI films before and after the May surgery, Dr. Neiman told us that she believed the tumor Dr. Kobrine said he had removed was still there. Another MRI later that day confirmed it to her satisfaction. Stunned and horrified, Stel and I discussed options with her. According to the recent MRI, the tumor was 2-3 cm larger than it had been at the time of Stel's first MRI in April, and Dr. Neiman told us she had explored gamma knife and had been told the tumor was too large. It became apparent very quickly that there were no options other than another surgery. Stel bravely decided to undergo a second operation, which was more risky because of the size of the tumor, on August 10th.

Wed Aug 11 1999 7:11 AM

Dear Kat, Sorry to send you bad news via e-mail, but I wanted you to know that Stel underwent a second brain operation yesterday. This is a result of what appears to be malpractice on the part of her previous surgeon. The nightmare we've been living since April has turned into a horror story. It appears that her previous surgeon did not remove all the tumor he could see, as he told us, but only did a biopsy. The tumor had been growing there ever since—all during radiation, which is ineffective against large masses. We discovered this after Stel had a seizure and was admitted to the hospital. Stel came through the operation yesterday well and her new surgeon said she believes she removed all of the (much larger) tumor that she could see. If that is the case, it will buy us a few months, but it grows fast and we have to find the next treatment that Stel can take to try to arrest its growth. Of course, since Stel already had the maximum safe radiation dose, she can't have that treatment now when it might be more effective. It's a devastating situation, but we're doing our best to keep going and keep hoping. She is in intensive care today. I'll let you know in a couple of days if she's in a room where she can receive calls. Love, Kay

Sun Aug 15 1999 10:42 AM

Dear Kat, Thanks for your message. Stel is out of intensive care now. She's had a rough time, and so have her cousin Bill and I, who have been at the hospital constantly. But yesterday she managed to talk to the doctor more than she's been able to talk before, although her throat is still extremely sore, and she still has a feeding tube down it. This morning she told me she wants "very cold pineapple juice," which doesn't sound good for a sore throat at all to me, but she's insistent she wants it, so I'm about to go off to get it. She's definitely getting better now, but still has no movement on her left side—except that when she was talking to the doctor yesterday, she was caught moving her left index finger a couple of times. A good sign, of course. I don't know how long she'll be in the hospital—probably another 4-5 days at least. Then the doctor wants to send her to the National Rehabilitation Hospital, where she can get intensive physical therapy.... I know Stel would want me to send you her good wishes. Thanks so much for keeping in touch. Love, Kay

Tue Aug 24 1999 6:38 AM

Dear George, I'm sorry to tell you (in confidence) that Stella has had a serious setback as a result of unbelievable malpractice on the part of her former neurosurgeon. She's been in the hospital for two weeks and just yesterday was transferred to a rehab unit where she'll need to do some intensive physical therapy to regain functionality on her left side. Her new doctor thinks that she'll be walking well enough to go home in no more than a couple of weeks. She's only now getting to the point where she can talk on the phone. PLEASE DON'T SAY ANYTHING TO THE FAMILY. STEL DID NOT WANT THEM TO KNOW UNTIL SHE COULD TALK TO THEM HERSELF.

As for the Crete property, Stel did everything she could to notify the architects that she wanted to get the property registered as soon as possible. She's, of course, in no shape now to follow up, so if you could take that on and try to ride herd on it, I know she'd be immensely grateful. I'd also suggest, George, that you might want to plan a trip to visit Stel before too long. She's got a terrible struggle ahead of her once she regains her ability to walk, and your support and love would undoubtedly mean a lot. I wish I could send you better news. Thanks for your concern and help. Best wishes, Kay

Wed Aug 25 1999 7:32 AM

Dear Fred, Just wanted to let you know that Stel has been moved to a rehab facility in Gaithersburg. She's made significant strides in the last 2-3 days in moving her left arm and leg and, in fact, yesterday insisted she was going to walk to the bathroom. With the help of her cousin and me, she took about twelve steps, which is phenomenal. Her goal at the moment is to walk well enough with some support to be able to get up the ten steps to our apartment so that she can come home. Her program of physical and occupational therapy starts today and I wouldn't be surprised to see her walking pretty well within a week or two. Kay

Thu Aug 26 1999 6:52AM

Dear Fred, Thanks so much for the donated leave, the prayers, good thoughts, etc. Stel amazed her trainers yesterday with her strength and determination. She wants to get out of these institutions and come home, which would be the greatest psychological boost she could have—and for me, too. I'll keep you posted on progress. Kay

Wed Sep 01 1999 3:45AM

Dear Edie, I've been intending to get in touch with you for the last couple of weeks, but just don't have the time these days for everything I need and want to do. Can't take the time now for a long message but I wanted you to know that Stel is making incredible progress every day in moving her arm and leg and yesterday even walked with a four-pronged cane across a large room. She wants to come home, and I want that too. She's got to get herself functional as soon as possible because we have little time to move on to other therapies. Even though the tumor was completely removed this time—the surgeon showed us on the MRI after the surgery—it's likely growing back quickly and we've got to find a way to stop it. I'm now on leave without pay but am hoping to get several weeks of paid leave through federal leave-sharing. Beyond that, I'll just have to take a leave of absence. There's no way I can, or want to, work in the foreseeable future. Stel is the first priority. Sorry the news is so bad. However, as I said, Stel is an inspiration every day—brave, strong, determined to beat the odds. Until later, Kay

Sun Sep 05 1999 4:31 PM

Dear Edie, We will be seeing a malpractice attorney. The man is a menace, despite his reputation. Stel is brave and strong and astonished her therapists at the rehab place with her rapid progress from hardly moving anything on her left side to walking well enough with a cane to come home yesterday. She still has a lot of work to do with home therapy to regain full functioning in her arm and leg, but she's done remarkably well. We'll move on to the next steps soon and do everything we can to beat the odds on this horrible tumor. It's all terrifying, but we're dealing with it day by day in the best way we can. Thanks for your love and good wishes, Kay

NOTE: We did file a malpractice suit against Dr. Kobrine, along with another plaintiff, a woman I met through the BT List who had had a similar experience with him in July 1998 and had a second craniotomy to remove most of the tumor four months after her first surgery with Kobrine. Fortunately, her tumor was slow-growing and since her second operation in November 1998, she has done well. There was a third patient of Dr. Kobrine's that we learned of, a man who Kobrine operated on in April 1999, one month before Stella, who said Kobrine had not removed all the tumor he said he had. Initially, we thought he would join the lawsuit, but ultimately he decided not to. I won't elaborate further here on the ins and outs of that litigation, which could take a book itself, but will simply say that we had the not-infrequent problem of finding expert witnesses willing to testify against another doctor (we did find one—on the West Coast) and for various other reasons, including a lawyer who got cold feet as we moved closer to trial, I decided to dismiss the suit in November 2002. I still believe that Stel and the other plaintiff suffered needlessly and underwent second operations because Dr. Kobrine failed to do what he said he did. I believe Stel's quality, and probably her quantity, of life was affected adversely by what he failed to do. Her second surgeon would have testified to that. I will be glad to speak privately to any reader who desires more information.

Sun Sep 12 1999 9:34 PM

Hi everyone [on BT List], My name is Kay Loveland. My partner of thirty years, Stelyani (Stel) Sandris, was diagnosed with a brain tumor in April '99. On May 6th, she had a craniotomy and the surgeon—a man with a big reputation and long experience—told us he had removed all the tumor that he could see, which he said was a good walnut size, from the right frontal lobe. He also wrote that in his operative report. Ten days after the surgery, he called to tell her that the tumor had been lost and therefore only the tiny biopsy sample taken during the operation existed for testing. That test had come back as a GBM. However, he didn't think the tumor looked "as ugly" as the worst tumors usually do, and that gave us a lot of hope. Thirteen days after the surgery, Stel had a second MRI. We were disturbed to see that the report stated there was a mass substantially larger than the mass before the surgery, but the surgeon assured us that this was per-fectly normal swelling and that everything looked just as it should. He also assured us that he and the oncologist he was referring Stel to would "honcho" Stel's case and "do everything" they could and they "could beat it."

With the same MRI report in front of him, the oncologist said there were "enhancing areas" on the MRI that indicated activity. But he spoke always of a "small lesion" in the past tense. Stel went through 6 1/2 weeks of radiation. The radiation oncologist also spoke of a small tumor in the past tense and never indicated that she was radiating a fairly large tumor. We both believed what was being radiated were the microscopic seedlings left behind after the visible tumor had been removed. Stel went through radiation well, as she had come through the surgery. The oncologist spoke effusively of how exceptionally well she was doing. A week after radiation ended, Stel began to feel weakness in her left side that she hadn't felt since right after the surgery. We both thought this might be a delayed effect of radiation, which I had read could happen, or that it was attributable to radiation swelling and the fact that she had been on only 4 mg of Decadron throughout radiation. At the end of the second week after radiation, on Friday, August 6th—three months to the day from the previous surgery—Stel had a seizure, the first full-fledged one she had had. It was 10:30 at night. She was perfectly lucid but unable to move her left side. I called the emergency number for the surgeon. He called back within five minutes. Stel and I were both on the phone and told him she had had a seizure and asked what he wanted to do. He was very cold and rude. He said he hadn't seen Stel in weeks, didn't know what was going on, and advised she should go to an emergency room. I then called 911 and she was taken to the local ER.

After a CT scan revealed excessive swelling on the brain, the ER doctor called the surgeon and told him that his patient needed to be admitted to the hospital. He thought the surgeon would want her to go where he practiced. The surgeon said he wouldn't take her in transfer. Not believing his ears, the ER doctor asked whether the surgeon agreed that she should be admitted to the hospital. The surgeon said yes, but he wouldn't do it. The outraged ER doctor then told Stel and me that the surgeon was a jerk and we should get a new neurosurgeon. We immediately asked for a young woman surgeon who had given us a second opinion. In the middle of the night I went home and got the MRI films and reports so she could see them immediately. When she came to see Stel the next morning she said she suspected that the surgeon had not removed the tumor as he said he had. She noted the post-op MRI report about the larger mass and said that did not refer to edema. An MRI taken the next day confirmed to her satisfaction that the tumor was still there, now more than twice as large as it was in April, and significantly larger than it was after the operation in May.

After we recovered from the shock and discussed options with the surgeon, Stel decided to have a second craniotomy the next day. She came through it okay, but with greater weakness on her left side than before. After sixteen days in the hospital, she was transferred to a rehab facility. When she went in, she could move her left index finger and wiggle her toes on her left foot. After eight days of physical and occupational therapy, she walked out with a four-pronged cane. She's now getting home therapy and making progress every day, but she tires very easily. We saw her new oncologist and surgeon this week. She will have another MRI in a couple of weeks so we can see where we are before she goes into further treatment. The oncologist is recommending six rounds of PCV with thalidomide thrown in 6-9 months down the road. I'd appreciate anybody's thoughts about that regimen, and about other drugs you'd throw in the mix. I'm interested in Poly ICLC; not sure about thalidomide as opposed to tamoxifen and temozolomide; also SU101 and marimastat. And what about melatonin, hydrazine sulfate, and Poly-MVA? Finally, what are your views on Dr. Burzynski's treatment in Houston? Also, I'd be interested in knowing where I can get Jeanne Wallace's nutrition protocol.

Sorry for the very long introduction, but don't know how to make any shorter the tale of our journey from nightmare to horror story. We will be pursuing action against the first surgeon, at least to try to stop him from doing the same thing to others. I'm excited to find the BT List and all the good information I've received in just one day. Problem is, how am I going to have time to read and digest everything. Anyway…I look forward to your responses.

Kay, partner of Stel

Mon Sep 13 1999 10:57 AM

Dear Kay, I was horrified to read your account of the way the doctors dealt with Stel, but I can't say I was surprised. My own experiences since being diagnosed with a GBM have not increased my regard for the medical profession. I often wonder how the doctors get away with such conduct. It's good that you shared your story with the BRAINTMR List. It's surprising how many people on the List have unquestioning trust in their medical team, and are reluctant to ask hard questions, doublecheck what the doctors tell them, or "push back" when necessary. Posts like yours will help them understand the need to be more aggressive to get proper care. Good luck, and best wishes to you and Stel. Steve (51, GBM dx 1/98, subtotal resection 1/98, radiation 2/97-3/98, recurrence 4/98, Temodar (12 rounds) 4/98-3/99, recurrence 4/99, gross total resection 4/99, BCNU (2 rounds) 5/99-8/99)

Mon Sep 13 1999 11:14 AM

Hello Kay, I had an eerily similar experience with my first neurosurgeon. He insisted he had gotten all of tumor and ridiculed me when I questioned him about the mass that still showed clearly in the post-op MRI (six weeks after surgery). He said what I saw was just swelling from surgery and to wait and see, to come back in three months and he could put a shunt in to drain fluid at that time, if necessary. I wasn't comfortable with this approach because I couldn't square what I could see with my own eyes with what he was telling me. So I spent two months getting second, third, fourth opinions. Each one said there was residual tumor that needed to be removed. I finally selected a new neurosurgeon who did my second surgery, four months after the first. Much better outcome after second surgery. No one facing such life-threatening circumstances should have to go through this. I'd like to discuss in more detail with you, if you have time and energy to do so. Thanks, Robin [She became the other plaintiff in our lawsuit.]

Sat Sep 25 1999 9:12 AM

Dear Stella, A few minutes ago, while browsing the Internet I brought up the web page of the Greek Embassy and was presented with the news of the "Cacoyannis Film Retrospective" which is to take place on Dec 4-18 at the National Gallery. At this point I must presume that, with all your health problems, you still managed to pull the Cacoyannis project through at the National Gallery. Wow!!!! Much luv, George

Tue Sep 28 1999 7:36 AM

Dear George, We didn't respond sooner because Stel and I went to a brain tumor conference in New Jersey on Saturday and Sunday. It was worthwhile. Stel is doing fine. Improving her walking every day. She had her first MRI since right after the surgery on Friday. We're nervously awaiting an appointment with her surgeon tomorrow to find out what it tells us. On Monday, Oct. 4, we have an appointment with a neuro-oncologist at Johns Hopkins. Soon thereafter, Stel will have to make a decision on what next. It's a very difficult question, given that no doctor will be able to tell her that one treatment works significantly better than another, and there are so many different drugs and other types of treatments being tried. But the doctor at Hopkins should have a handle on the most promising possibilities. Re the Cacoyannis program, Stel did, in fact, pull the program together and will be excited to know that the Embassy is promoting it. Best, Kay

Wed Oct 6 1999 8:57 AM

Mary, Stel and I saw Dr. Grossman at Hopkins on Monday. He told Stel her recent scan of 9/24 looks "great." He wants the neuro-pathologist there to review the pathology slides of the tumor to see whether a lot of what looked like "live" tumor on the scan taken before surgery was actually "dead" tumor from radiation. Once they have a look at the slides, he said he'd have a better idea of what, if anything, he would recommend as the next step. He indicated that at Hopkins they advocate watching and waiting and that Stel should get monthly scans. When tumor regrowth is confirmed, then he would recommend chemo. We asked him about a stereotactic radiosurgery boost and he was quite negative about that as well as a couple of other things I'd heard Dr. Selker from U of Pitt talk about at the brain tumor conference. I liked him very much, but I'm wondering if maybe the approach at Hopkins is rather conservative. I'd appreciate having your assessment of him. Of course, Stel and I are happy that the recent scan looks pretty much as it did right after surgery—there's a little residual enhancement that no one can tell what it is. I just don't want to wait around hoping for miracles rather than doing something that might retard regrowth even more than it is apparently retarded now. Best wishes, Kay

Sun Oct 10 1999 9:32 PM

Dear Renata, A lot has happened since we last communicated. For now, I'll say our spirits are pretty good, given everything we've been through, but there's a very hard road ahead. Fortunately, Stel's most recent MRI scan showed no regrowth of the tumor yet, and her doctor advocates watching and waiting before starting further treatment with chemotherapy or focused radiation. We're happy she's doing so well right now, but knowing the aggressive nature of this horrible tumor, we're not going to rely on just one doctor's opinion of what to do. People with these beasts in their brains get input from different doctors and try to make sense out of the differing recommendations. There is no treatment at this point that any doctor can tell you is better than any other, and there are a lot of different drugs being tested, as well as other procedures being experimented with, so it makes decisions extremely difficult to make. It's really awful, but all one can do is learn as much as possible and make the best decisions one can, and if the treatments chosen don't seem to have any positive effect fairly quickly, move on to something else. It's terrifying, horrifying, and exhausting, but some people do beat the very bad odds, and we don't see why Stel shouldn't be one of those people.

I've been unable to work since August 6th. So far I'm able to use about 300 hours of leave time that has been donated to me from coworkers and other federal employees. I'm hoping I'll get still more donated time. When that runs out, I'll have to take an unpaid leave of absence. Given the totally unpredictable nature of these tumors, I find it hard to envision when I could possibly try to do any work, even part time. Right now, the only job I can do or want to do is to help Stel get the best treatment she can. Nothing else matters. In addition to the focus on Stel's health and treatment, we're also talking to lawyers about filing a malpractice lawsuit against Stel's first surgeon for failing to remove the tumor as he said he did. We've found out that he did the same thing to at least two other people in the last year, and we all feel we've got to try to stop him. No telling how many others he's done it to or will do it to. It's bizarre and horrifying.

I wish the news could be better from here—but it could be far worse, as well. As we tell all our friends, just keep all those good thoughts, good wishes, good vibes coming Stel's way. She needs all of them. We're hoping that Stel will be able by next June to go to spend a month or so at a Swedish friend's summer house on a Baltic island outside of Stockholm. That's been a dream of hers for a long time and I pray she'll be able to do it—but who knows what we'll be dealing with at that point, which is an eternity in tumor time. God willing that she gets there, we'd love to see you there. Let's all visualize a happy reunion during the summer solstice in the Baltic. Love, Kay

Sun Oct 10 1999 9:42 PM

Dear Karla, Sorry I haven't gotten back to you sooner. I had major computer problems, which I really needed on top of everything else I'm trying to deal with. Anyway, we went to see a neuro-oncologist at Johns Hopkins last Monday and he said Stel's MRI looks "great." In other words, there's no firm evidence of regrowth right now. There is a small area of residual enhancement that can't be defined—could be "post-operative change," as they say, or dead cells from radiation, or regrowth. It's small and he advocates watching and waiting and not doing other treatment yet. He wants her to get MRIs every month or so and when (I wish I could say if) it begins growing again, then he would propose a chemotherapy regimen. We were very happy that he was so positive about Stel's situation now—he thinks she's doing very well, which she is—but know that we can't rest on our laurels. People with these kinds of tumors get a variety of opinions from different doctors and try to sort out what seems the best thing to do. No doctor can really tell you that. I'm going to send Stel's scans off to at least a couple of other doctors to see what they think would be the right course to take now. I'm not sure that waiting for the tumor to come back is the best thing to do, even though this doctor is an expert in the field. Other experts would probably have different opinions. It's a terrible situation to be in and it's awful to have to make these decisions, but what else can one do?

At any rate, Stel is gaining strength every day and is more and more herself. We're hoping she'll be strong enough in another ten days or so to go to visit friends in the Chicago area, and also go to a clinic we had been planning to go to before her second operation. Her spirits are good and we're determined to do everything we can to help her beat the odds. So keep your good thoughts, prayers, etc. coming this way. It's all overwhelming, but we just keep plugging. Love, Kay

Mon Oct 11 1999 8:54 PM

Dear Karla, I'll definitely pass your hug along. We've made our plans to go to Chicago on the 19th, returning on the 27th. Stel has an appointment with the medical center there on the 21st. It's not an alternative center but is an integrative one—in other words, they make use of the best information about nutrition and other alternative treatments as well as conventional. They will do a thorough evaluation of Stel's situation and give us their best thoughts. We're looking forward to spending time with our friends there, too. I just hope the trip isn't too exhausting for Stel. Climbing on and off crowded airplanes is tiring in itself. I'll let you know how it goes. Love, Kay

Thu Nov 04 1999 11:47 PM

Dear Robin, We talked to Stel's surgeon about her MRI this week [Nov. 1]. The news wasn't as good as last time, but nowhere near the worst, either. She said there is slightly increased enhancement in a couple of peripheral areas, and some increased swelling. She thinks this indicates tumor growth, though others might disagree. In her opinion, Stel should decide on the next step in treatment in 2-3 weeks. We're in accord on this since we're not comfortable with just watching and waiting to be sure what's going on. We'll see her neuro-oncologist at Hopkins next week and find out what, if anything, he would suggest at this stage. She's also been approved for a stereotactic radiation procedure in Chicago [at the Chicago Institute of Neurosurgery and Neuroresearch (CINN)] and is leaning heavily in the direction of doing that soon, although I know the neuro-onc will be against that when we talk to him. It's so wonderful to have so much consensus about these deadly serious matters. I'll sign off for now. Hope you're well. Kay

Fri Nov 05 1999 12:04 AM

Dear Vanessa, We'll miss you at dinner. If plans change, please feel free to barge in at the last minute. I'll let you know where we decide to go.

We had somewhat less good news yesterday than the time before, but not really bad news. Bad news would have been that the beast is barrelling ahead, undaunted by radiation, surgery, etc. That doesn't seem to be the case yet, and we'll do everything we can to see that it isn't the case. We had excellent news today about a blood test Stel took in Chicago for her immune system—something you would think would be standard, but it isn't. It indicated, among other things, that her natural killer cell activity was 92 out of 100. The woman who called us about the results called them "wonderful" and a "great scenario." The nutritionist we're now consulting with [Jeanne Wallace] said it was unheard of for someone battling what Stel is and in her age range to score so high. So I guess we've been doing something right with all the stuff I've been shoving down her gullet during these months and now that we have a real regimen worked out by someone who knows a lot more about this than I do, I think her immune system will be boosted even more. So she'll be in excellent shape for whatever comes next. That may be stereotactic radiosurgery in Chicago soon and then some chemo.

Anyway, Stel would love to read your paper any time you can give it to her, and we'll look forward to hearing about your travels as soon as you're able. Love, Kay

Thu Nov 11 1999 5:14 PM

Dear Ann, I've been meaning to write you a note ever since we got back to send you Stel's and my thanks for the lovely few hours at your house. It was great to see you and pleasant to spend time in your nice sunny rooms and garden. Stel's still doing fine. We're now facing the awful problem of trying to decide what to do next based on totally conflicting medical opinions. It's all a crapshoot and not a task I would wish on my worst enemy. We've tentatively scheduled a date—Dec. 2nd—for Stel to have a focused radiation procedure at CINN in Chicago. However, her neuro-oncologist is completely against this and has recommended the most conservative chemo approach possible. I'm now trying to get a couple of other opinions about the radiosurgery. Whatever we decide on, we need to do it within the next three weeks and get Stel started as it appears the beast is rearing its ugly head again—ever so slightly—inside her brain. It's terribly frightening, but we're plugging ahead as best we can. I hope we'll have a chance to visit your house in Guadalajara one of these days. We'll keep that as one of our good visions to ward off the demons. I'll let you know for sure if and when we'll be back in Chicago. Love, Kay

Tue Nov 23 1999 8:35 AM

Dear Mary, Stel and I are sending our best thoughts to you and your sister today. It's awful going through these MRIs. I'd be interested to know how your sister is tolerating CPT-11 (if it's working). I was a little taken aback when Dr. Grossman recommended only BCNU for Stel. Did he make such a conservative recommendation to your sister first? He is also very much against stereotactic radiosurgery for Stel, but we've decided to go ahead with it in Chicago, where they can use the Peacock for a one-shot boost and they've done hundreds of tumors and tumor cavities that are larger than most places seem to be willing to do. Our local oncologist and surgeon think it makes sense to do it. So, we'll go to Chicago on November 30th and the procedure will be on December 2nd. If everything goes as it's supposed to, Stel will be released on December 3rd, we'll see friends on the weekend and return home on Dec. 5th. After that, I think we'll go to Richmond to see Dr. [Randall] Merchant about Poly ICLC, and I'm going to contact Dr. [Henry] Friedman at Duke, too, for his recommendations. Our local oncologist also disagrees with Dr. Grossman about using only BCNU. She would opt for PCV with thalidomide later because she thinks the multiple drug approach is better. I do, too, but am not convinced we shouldn't go for a mix of newer drugs attacking the cells in different ways rather than the standard PCV. Anyway, we look forward to hearing that your sister's scan today looks super. All the best, Kay

Tue Nov 23 1999 8:39 AM

Dear Dr. Friedman, I'm writing on behalf of my partner, Stella Sandris, who was diagnosed with a GBM in the right frontal lobe in May. She has had two craniotomies (the second in August). All visible tumor was removed. She's been in rehab and recuperation since that time because of substantial weakness on her left side, but is doing pretty well now. She had an MRI on 9/24 which Dr. Grossman at Johns Hopkins said looked "great." He said we should watch and wait. Stel's second post-op MRI was on 11/1. There is a slight increase in enhancement in two places along the periphery and a little additional swelling in the left frontal lobe. Stel's surgeon and Dr. Grossman think this indicates tumor growth. Dr. Grossman recommended two rounds of BCNU and then a scan to see if it's working. He was not in favor of stereotactic radiosurgery. However, we have talked at length to Dr. [Tomasz] Helenowski at CINN and the committee there has approved Stel for the procedure, which we've decided to do on December 2nd. Our local oncologist is in agreement with this course. She then recommends that Stel start a course of PCV in about a month after the procedure. She would throw thalidomide into the mix down the line, assuming PCV is working.

Neither Stel nor I are convinced that BCNU or PCV are the ways to go. We believe hitting the tumor with different drugs, and some of the newer ones, probably makes more sense. We're also interested in Poly ICLC and have been in touch with Dr. Merchant about that. We'd like the benefit of your consultation as well. I think we'll be able to travel to Richmond and Durham in the early part of December. We'll look forward to hearing from you. Thanks, Kay Loveland

Tue Nov 23 1999 9:11 AM

To Kay Loveland—An on-site consultation in December is a great idea—we would use other agents rather than PCV or straight BCNU. I need the records sent to me (all surgeries, path reports, RT summary, radiosurgery, the most recent MRI, and the path slides). Henry [Friedman]

Wed Nov 24 1999 12:08 AM

Dear Mary, Thanks for your message. I am interested to hear about Dr. Grossman's approach with your sister—offering her experimental possibilities—because I was very surprised he didn't outline such possibilities for Stel. When I asked why he recommended BCNU, he said it is effective for a significant minority of patients and he didn't want to fail to try something that might work for Stel just because it's a drug that's been around for a long time. I suppose I could have raised more questions than I did, but he seemed so certain about taking the BCNU route and I guess I was unprepared for that. I did ask about Poly ICLC and he said, "well, it's experimental." At any rate, I don't think we're going to go the one drug route. Re the radiosurgery, everyone we've talked to except Grossman favors it, so he is in the minority among those we've polled. (I'm especially glad the procedure will be done with the Peacock.) I'll definitely let you know how it goes for her. All fingers and toes are crossed. Here's to a happy Thanksgiving. Kay

Wed Nov 24 1999 12:29 AM

Dear Dr. Friedman, Thanks for your response. I'll get all documentation off to you after our return from Chicago on Dec. 5th when we'll have latest MRI, etc. If Stel's feeling up to it, I'd like to go to Richmond and Duke by December 15th. Kay Loveland

Thu Nov 25 1999 9:29 AM

Dear Mary, I'm sorry to hear about your sister's scan. As you know I wouldn't take the word of Dr. Grossman or others at JH about whether radiosurgery would be an option for her. Stel's tumor is also described by Grossman as "too diffuse" for the procedure. The doctors at the CINN don't think so. We've talked to Dr. Helenowski, who will be doing the procedure, three times at length—twice on phone calls since we returned from Chicago—and he says he's done scores, if not hundreds, of tumors like Stel's and they believe that, overall, they achieve a median extension of time of 3-6 months. Of course, he can't say how Stel will respond and we know there are some risks—particularly swelling and necrosis—but Helenowski believes those risks are minimal, at least the first time this procedure is done. We're impressed with all the people we've dealt with there. I asked Helenowski why they would do things like this that most other places would say shouldn't or couldn't be done. He said the others probably don't want to spend the money because it is more time consuming, but the doctors at CINN are committed to trying to help patients others might not help. That sounds too good to be true, but after having talked to him and the nurses there several times, I believe him. Also, when we went to the Keith Block Clinic in Chicago, which takes a holistic approach to treating cancer, and mentioned that we had an appointment with Helenowski, they said that was good because they usually refer brain tumor patients to CINN. The other thing that I'm impressed with there is that they have three different ways of doing radiosurgery and they're going to use the Peacock machine for Stel's procedure because it is good for "diffuse" tumors. The Peacock is about the most sophisticated machine around right now and can be targeted much more precisely than any other machines. We're scared and worried that Stel will have some side effects from this, but believe it's worth the risks. The mother of another person on the list had it done with the Peacock about eight months ago and has had no problems (and clear MRIs) for several months now.

In early December we're planning to talk with Dr. Randall Merchant at the Virginia Medical College in Richmond about the Poly ICLC trial, and also with Dr. Friedman at Duke, who I'm sure will have other ideas for Stel. I'll keep you posted on those.

It was Dr. Robert Selker from U. of Pitt who spoke at the N.J. brain tumor conference about chemosensitivity testing, as well as "customizing" treatment for each tumor. They do radiosurgery there, too. I think he's worth getting in touch with. He also indicated that the insertion of the radioactive pellets was an option he thinks is effective. I know if Stel, god forbid, has to undergo a third surgery, it will be for more than just removing tumor. Something is going to be inserted.[4]

Anyway, I hope your Thanksgiving Day is as enjoyable as you can make it. As long as your sister wants to fight this beast, I think the key is just to keep looking and talking to different doctors in different places. As they say, they do have different "philosophies" about how to deal with this horrible "octopus," as Stel says. If you want to talk at any time, please call us. We'll be back from Chicago on December 5th. Stel has a film program that she planned for the National Gallery starting on December 4th. The following weekend, December 11th, she is supposed to introduce the filmmaker. She's very nervous about whether she'll be able to. Keep your fingers crossed that she can. It would be a shame, after she's managed to pull this all together during this frightful year, if she couldn't. All the best to you, Kay

Sat Nov 27 1999 9:10 AM

Dear Karla, Thanks for your Thanksgiving greetings. We had a lovely Thanksgiving with some friends at a country house in Virginia. Stel enjoyed the company and the food, as did I. Unfortunately, for the last couple of weeks, Stel hasn't been doing as well as she was with her balance and walking. She's been on Decadron since Nov. 10th and we've varied the dosage anywhere from 10 mg to 4 mg a

---

4.   After Stel's second surgery, when I got my wits about me, I asked her surgeon why she hadn't disussed implanting chemo wafers. She said she was worried about infection and implanting wafers might increase the danger of complications. Dr. Neiman had been infuriated to find that, three months after the first surgery, Stel's incision, which she would have to use for the second surgery, was still inflamed and tender, which greatly increased the risk of infection. (When we had asked about the scabs on the incision three weeks earlier, the oncologist had told us it looked "perfect." We accepted his word for it.)

day. At 10, she's seemed to be okay. Yesterday, at 8 mg she did well later in the day and her balance seemed much better. We took a walk in the morning and she kept leaning back and taking small steps. But, when I put my arm around her shoulders and walk with her, she can keep up with my stride. Anyway, as I said, she seemed much better in terms of her balance last night, but ironically, she fell for the first time in the bathroom. I think she slipped on the bath mat under her feet that I've tried to keep her from using for that very reason. At any rate, although she hit with a terrible thud, she seems to have escaped relatively unharmed (she realized this morning her ribs on her left side are sore but she doesn't seem to be in any significant pain so, hopefully, she didn't crack or break one). I'm worried about this backward-leaning walk and the need to keep the Decadron up to try to deal with it.

We're still planning to go to Chicago on November 30th for the stereotactic radiosurgery procedure, but with some trepidation. I hope to god it doesn't make the swelling significantly worse. I hate the thought of her having to be on big doses of Decadron for weeks to come. We did get another opinion from San Francisco about radiosurgery and chemo protocols and they were, surprisingly to me, just about as conservative as the doctor at Johns Hopkins. They wouldn't do radiosurgery on Stel because of the diffuseness of the tumor. However, the doctor who called said he had been at Chicago before going to SF and knew their work. It's "just" a difference in philosophy. These diametrically opposed philosophies about BT treatments are crazy-making. He would go with BCNU or Temozolomide, or maybe high-dose CPT-11. With these two doctors recommending against radiosurgery, we've felt it necessary to talk two more times on the phone with Dr. Helenowski in Chicago about questions raised. We also talked to our local oncologist who favors the radiosurgery and PCV thereafter, and to Stel's surgeon who also felt it made sense to go ahead with it. Helenowski has satisfied our questions as much as it's possible and, a significant factor in my view, is that he will be using the Peacock for Stel so that the radiation can be very precisely targeted. All the friends we've bounced the pros and cons off of say it sounds like the right thing to do now. So-o-o-o, we're keeping all fingers and toes crossed and trudging ahead. I'll let you know how it goes. Love, Kay

Tue Dec 07 1999 6:41 AM

Dear Friends, Stel came through a grueling 12+ hour day of the radiosurgery procedure (over eight hours of it with the metal headframe screwed on her head) like a champ but had an unanticipated seizure the next morning. Since she couldn't function well at all and, in fact, couldn't walk, she wasn't released on Friday morning as originally planned. Fortunately, by Saturday morning she was doing better and was able to walk with a lot of assistance. We went out to our friends and had a nice dinner with them and other Swedish friends on Saturday night. Sunday I managed, with some difficulty, to get us both back to the airport and on the plane and we were fortunate to have friends meet us at BWI. Stel is doing okay but her balance and walking are shakier than they were and she's having more word-finding difficulties than previously. I have no way of knowing whether this is transitory or permanent. She'll have a follow-up MRI in a month, but it will take longer to know how effective the radiation may have been. (The doctor in Chicago said it appeared the tumor was "taking off again" and felt it was good the procedure was being done now to "knock it back.") We'll see her surgeon today. Next week or the week after, if Stel is up to it and we can get appointments, we'll probably go to Richmond to talk to a doctor there about an immunotherapy trial and on down to Duke to consult with another doctor about chemo protocols other than those that have been recommended here. By the first of the year, she needs to make a decision about the next round of treatment.

Stel was still working over her introduction of Cacoyannis yesterday when she talked to Peggy and found out that he's under doctor's orders himself not to travel right now, so he won't be coming. It's a shame given all the effort Stel put into getting him here, but she agrees it's probably best since it takes all pressure off her. We'll probably still go to the screenings on Saturday. If you're in the mood for some good films, please come. Hope to see you there. I know Stel would love to talk to you before then. Kay

Wed Dec 08 1999 9:02 AM

Dear Linda, Stel got your message yesterday. I just wanted to tell you that things are not going well right now with her. Although she recovered her ability to walk after the seizure sufficiently so that I could manage to get her home, she's not functioning physically at the level she was. Her balance and walking are very shaky. Also, although she's fine for intellectual conversations and other interactions with friends, therapists, etc., she's unable to initiate or perform most daily functions, so I'm doing much more of that. Getting her out of the apartment and into the car has become an even more major effort. She saw her physical and occupational therapists yesterday and they agreed that she needs to go back to home therapy at this point. I'm deeply worried that the radiation procedure has caused her permanent damage but am trying to stay hopeful that the deterioration is only a transitory effect of the procedure and/or the seizure and/or the increased medication she's on. No doctor has an answer to that. I'm also hoping she'll be functioning well enough for me to take her down to Richmond next Monday and on to Duke on Tuesday/Wednesday. Given the situation, although it's disappointing that Cacoyannis can't come to D.C., Stel agrees it's probably better for her. She still wants to make the screenings on Saturday and may want to preview them when Peggy lets her know the schedule. Anyway, I just wanted to let you know more specifically what Stel's situation is at the moment. Until later, Kay

Wed Dec 08 1999 9:36 AM

Cathy, I wanted to let you know that Stel isn't doing as well as she was and is often unable to initiate mundane tasks like taking her pills, eating, etc. I'm having to help her much more than before the procedure and I'm very worried that she's suffered permanent damage, but I'm trying to stay hopeful that this is transitory effects of trauma to the brain or increased medications. I wish I could send you better news. Maybe in a couple of weeks, if the radiation has done its job, things will begin to improve, I'm hoping I'll be able to take her to Richmond and Duke next week for doctors' consultations before we make a final decision on what chemo to pursue. Unfortunately, from what the MRI in Chicago showed—before the procedure—the tumor appears to have begun to invade the left side of Stel's brain. We've got to throw all the ammo we can find at it. I'm heartbroken but do my best to keep a positive outlook. Stel is coping as well as possible, I think, with a horrible situation (although, as I tell her, not as bad as some I've read about who have improved). Until later, Kay

Wed Dec 08 1999 11:32 PM

Dear Mary, Thanks so much for your message and attachment. Stel is entirely responsible for the film program being offered at the National Gallery. She started working on it more than two years ago. Nice to see the word is being spread.

I wish I had better news to report after the radiosurgery procedure. Of course, time will tell whether it's been effective, and whether it's resulted in lasting deficits to Stel. What's most disturbing is that she's been completely unable to initiate anything since then—mostly just watches TV and I've had to feed her sometimes and nearly always pop pills down her throat to be sure they're taken. This wasn't the case before. She also takes no initiative in getting dressed and spends even more time with her toiletries than previously. It's very depressing and scary. And, of course, no one seems to be able to say whether this is due to the seizure she had the day after, the procedure, additional medications or whether it's transitory or permanent. She seems to be a little livelier tonight, so I'm hoping maybe she's coming out of the trance. But she's also more confused than she was, at least when she's talking to me. She can carry on perfectly lucid conversations with friends and therapists. We're going to see a neurologist tomorrow and, hopefully, he can sort some of this out. Needless to say, I'm beside myself—very upset and worried that we shouldn't have proceeded with this, but what can you do? Get all the information you can and make the best decision you can in this surreal world of complete unpredictability. I just pray Stel will become more herself with some time—and that the radiation did some real damage to the tumor. We have an appointment in Richmond on Monday afternoon to talk with Dr. Merchant, and I was trying to set something up at Duke for Tuesday or Wednesday. Now I don't know whether I can manage to get Stel there and whether she'll be up to it. But it's so important that we move on quickly now and make our decision about the next step.

I'm glad your sister seems to be doing pretty well. I'll be interested to know how she does on Temodar because that's one of the drugs I think we probably should be using immediately. Again, thanks for your good thoughts. Keep 'em coming. Kay

Wed Dec 08 1999 11:38 PM

Dear Linda, We talked to Peggy tonight and got the preview schedule for tomorrow and Friday. I doubt we'll make it. I'm taking Stel to a neurologist tomorrow and don't think we'll be able to manage two outings. (She seems to be a little livelier tonight, so I'm hoping maybe she's coming out of this trance she's been in.) Friday afternoon some friends are planning to come over, so that will cut into the time for the preview that day. But Stel will be at the Saturday screenings. Then we may be going to Richmond and Duke on Mon-Wed. Depends on whether I think it's manageable to drive down there with her. Love, Kay

NOTE: Because of her balance and cognitive problems, Stel's neurologist decided to put her in the hospital on December 9th so she could undergo some tests. I was glad he was taking a closer look at her but worried that she wouldn't be able to attend the screening of the program she had planned on the 11th, and even more, that I wouldn't be able to take her to Richmond and Duke at the beginning of the following week.

Mon Dec 13 1999 10:53 AM

Dear Carole, Stel was discharged from the hospital on Saturday and made a triumphant appearance at the screening of the Cacoyannis documentary that afternoon. It was a packed house.

They learned nothing new in the hospital. No on-going seizures. Swelling, but no assessment if it's much more than before the SR procedure. We'll probably know more next week when Stel gets another CT scan and we see the neurologist again. She's walking better and now has a rolling walker. Much brighter the last couple of days, and especially this morning. Still not initiating much, but a little. More herself, at any rate, to my relief. Hopefully Stel's brain is beginning to recover from the trauma, at least partially. We're leaving for Richmond shortly to see Dr. Merchant and then on to Duke tomorrow to see what Henry Friedman would recommend. Until later, Kay

Thu Dec 23 1999 1:24 AM

Dear Robin, Thanks for your message. I wish I could say the last few weeks have been good, but they haven't. We did go to Chicago, where Stel had SR on Dec. 2nd. We had talked to the doctor three times and asked every question we could think of about the likelihood of adverse side effects, etc., and had talked to other doctors who had conflicting opinions, and batted the pros and cons back and forth a dozen times before deciding to go ahead. From everything we could gather, the risk of serious side effects was minimal, but Stel apparently is in the small group who experience them. The day after the procedure, she had a seizure and was really unable to function well at all, couldn't even walk. Fortunately, she got better and we flew back to Maryland a couple of days later. But she's not functioning as well physically or cognitively as she was before the procedure. Her walking and balance are shakier, although she had been having some problems before we left. Even more upsetting to me, when we first came home for several days she was unable to initiate anything herself and I really had to do everything for her. Her brain was very scrambled up and she had a much harder time than before finding words and finishing sentences, etc. I was beside myself.

On Thursday and Friday last week, she was admitted to the hospital, where the neurologist did a CT scan and EEG to see if anything unusual was going on.

Nothing was. By Saturday, Stel had begun to improve enough that she was discharged and I was able to take her down to the National Gallery for the film program that she had planned over this year. And on Monday and Tuesday we drove down to Richmond to see Dr. Merchant and to Duke to see Dr. Friedman. We liked Friedman a lot and he's going to supervise this next phase. We liked Merchant, too, but Friedman isn't enthusiastic about the trial Merchant is running on Poly ICLC. Stel will start chemo this week with CCNU. In five weeks, she'll have an MRI and Friedman said he could tell enough from that to know whether it is being effective or not. If not, he'll switch her, probably, to Temodar. We like it that he will stay on top of this and, unlike Dr. Grossman at Johns Hopkins, won't wait twelve weeks (through two rounds of BCNU) before assessing effectiveness. Unfortunately, from everything we can gather, Stel's tumor is pretty fast-growing, and waiting twelve weeks seems unwise to us. Hopefully, the radiation will kick in and slow things down for a while, too, although Friedman had his doubts that it would be very effective. I'm hoping the fact that Stel seems to be improving daily indicates the radiation is having an effect. I'm worried, though, that she's not as functional as she was three weeks ago. She's going to start home PT and OT again next week. She had been going to out-patient sessions, but given her regression, home therapy seems more helpful now. I'm also worried that she's having problems with her writing, which she had for a while after surgery, and have got to see about some home speech therapy, too, and probably a visit to a neuro-psychologist as well. And I'm working on getting some home health care assistance to take some of the load off me.

As you can see, it's been a frantic and worrisome few weeks. I'm just grateful every day for the small improvements I see in Stel's ability to function. It's so painful to see her in this situation. Hope you have good holidays. All the best, Kay

Thu Dec 23 1999 1:46 AM

Dear Mary, Stel has improved on a daily basis, but still isn't back to where she was before the radiosurgery. What can you do? The odds for a treatment seem pretty good and you hope you're not in the minority who experience significant side effects. Unfortunately, it appears Stel probably was in that minority. But she's already made remarkable progress in pulling out of the funk she was in, and I pray that progress will continue with more home PT and OT. She also probably will need more cognitive assistance than she was getting before. At any rate, Stel was functioning well enough to go to the Cacoyannis screening on December

11th. The crowd was overflowing and, according to the woman who runs the film programs at the Gallery, the series was a huge success. Stel is happy that it's over and went well. After that weekend, we drove down to Richmond to see Randall Merchant and on to Duke to see Henry Friedman. Friedman is supervising the next phase. He recommended she start on CCNU this week. He saw no reason to give her BCNU intravenously, as Grossman advocated. In five weeks Stel will get a scan and he will decide whether to continue for another round or switch her to something else, probably Temodar.

Stel's been on Decadron since November 10th. She was having some walking problems that the doctor thought were related to swelling and so we played around with a dosage from 4 to 10 mg up until she had radiosurgery done on Dec. 2nd. At that time, they put her on 24 mg a day and she's been on a slow taper downward since then. She's now at 16 and, hopefully, will keep going down by 2 mg every four days until she's off it in mid-January. In addition to the steroid, she's on two anti-seizure meds—Tegretol and Depakote, the latter she has been taking since she had the seizure in Chicago on Dec. 3rd. So, how much of her lack of functioning is due to medications is anyone's guess, but given what you say your sister is experiencing, maybe a great deal is due to that. I'll keep you posted on Stel's progress and will keep good thoughts coming your way. Hope you have good holidays. Kay

Sat Dec 25 1999 8:45 AM

Dear Karla, Hope you're having a Merry Christmas. It's good to hear from you. Stel is doing pretty well right now, but not as well as she was before the radiosurgery procedure, back in October, early November. I was very worried a couple of weeks ago, and the doctor put her in the hospital for a couple of days to observe her and do tests. Didn't find anything notable, but while she was in the hospital, she began to improve and has continued to do so for the last week. I'm very relieved, even though she's still not functioning as well as she was. Stel will begin chemo this weekend by taking a couple of pills of one of the standard drugs. Then she'll wait five weeks, have an MRI, and if the doctor thinks it's having a beneficial effect, she'll take another round of the pills in 5-6 weeks. The "success" rate with this drug is around 30%, which is the highest of any drug for trying to treat these horrible tumors. If Stel has any luck, which so far has eluded her, she'll be one of the 30%. Unfortunately, her tumor has begun to regrow at a couple of points around the periphery of where the original tumor was removed in August (and, distressingly, into the dominant side of her brain). We're hoping that the radiation she had will stunt its growth for several months and that the chemo will be effective in holding it back for more months. If this chemo doesn't appear to be working in five weeks, the doctor will go on to another. There are many drugs and other treatments in trials going on and it seems likely that within 2-3 years something better than what there is now will come along. The goal is to keep Stel going until that point. It's a horrible, terrifying battle, but she's fighting hard and her doctor was amazed when she saw her this past week at how well she looked and is doing despite everything. She was especially impressed that Stel had made it to her program and went on the trip to Duke.

The brain tumor world is surreal and completely unpredictable. I'm on a brain tumor e-mail list and it's clear that everyone dealing with these horrendous beasts is trying to cope with unimaginable situations. The doctors really know so little about these tumors and, after you've had surgery and standard radiation, there is absolutely no consensus among them as to what is the best treatment to pursue. We had directly conflicting opinions from several doctors when we were trying to decide about the intensive radiation procedure. Ultimately, patients just have to gather as much information as they can and make their own decisions as well as they can. It's not a reassuring feeling.

As for my situation, fortunately, due to the generosity of coworkers, friends, and some people I don't know, I've been able to keep a partial paycheck coming in for the past many weeks and think I'll be able to stretch it out into February. When the donated time runs out, I'll have to decide what to do. I'm hoping that Stel will do well on the chemo and not have bad side effects (low white blood counts and nausea are the two main ones) and that things will calm down a bit so that perhaps I can do some part-time work at home. So far, there's no way I could have focused on any work and, given the unpredictability of the situation, that may be a pipe dream, but I hope I'll be able to find some time for that in January-February. However, I also hope Stel will be up to traveling during that time so that we can go to Phoenix and stay at Dana's for ten days or so. It would be a good break for us. But who knows whether that will be feasible. (If we do, we'll need some help to fly out there. It's extremely difficult trying to fly with Stel now since she has to be in a wheelchair in the airport. I nearly went crazy getting to and from Chicago.)

You asked about the seizure Stel had. Unfortunately, seizures are a common experience for people who've had brain tumors and surgery. Many people have them quite frequently. So far, Stel hasn't experienced that—a lot depends on where the tumor is located—but she's now had three seizures—one in August when we took her to the ER, one after the surgery and one after the radiation procedure this month. The last two have been "brain" seizures in that they weren't visible to anyone looking, but their effect is to make her unresponsive for about a day and, more long-lasting, they've exacerbated the weakness on her left side. She's now taking two different anti-seizure medications. Emotionally, Stel is remarkable. She still has her sense of humor and irony and often laughs at her inability to do things she could otherwise do. She can see the absurdity of the situation even in the midst of the nightmare. So she laughs a lot, cries some, too, but in general we're trying to live our lives as close to normal as we can—visiting with friends, watching movies, talking about politics, eating good food, enjoying each other's company, as we always have. I'm laughing a lot, too, keeping as light a touch as possible with Stel, but it's very hard to see her in this situation, and frightening and depressing to confront the future. So far, I've been able to remain pretty upbeat about everything and keep focused on the positive and the bits of progress Stel makes daily.

As for what sustains us: Neither of us is religious. Our faith is in our own profound caring for each other. As I said, laughing helps a lot (we're renting funny movies—just wish there were more; so many of the more recent ones don't elicit a chuckle from us), and seeing the irony in otherwise depressing situations. I've always been a person who just tries to deal with what confronts me as well as I can, and that's what I'm doing here. There's a great deal to be done each day and I keep focused on getting it done and trying to think ahead to what I need to do tomorrow and next week to try to affect things in a positive way, and to try to anticipate what needs Stel may have. As everyone trying to cope with brain tumors says, it's best to try to take things a day at a time. We have today and it's a good one, so enjoy it for all it's worth, treasure and savor it. If tomorrow's a bad day, it may be followed by a better day. That's about all one can do. I'm very grateful for your interest and caring. Hope to talk to you later today. Love, Kay

Sat Dec 25 1999 9:10 AM

Dear Ann, We drove down to Richmond and on to Duke almost two weeks ago. It actually turned out to be an enjoyable trip because the weather was lovely. It was hard dealing with Stel all by myself, but not as hard as traveling by plane. We liked the doctor at Duke, and he is now supervising the next phase of treatment.

As I told you, Stel has had significant problems since the radiosurgery procedure. Given the deficits she's suffered from it, I pray it will at least have some beneficial effect, buy her several months of time by stunting the tumor's growth. It's hard for me to believe it won't with the huge radiation dose that zapped the tumor area.

Yesterday, I had to take her to the ER because of swollen glands at the base of her neck on each side. She had no fever or any other symptoms of infection. Of course, being Christmas Eve, her doctor was not reachable so the only way to get attention was to go to the ER and then have them get in touch with her partner who was covering over this weekend. After a couple of hours, they decided to let Stel go and said if the swelling gets worse or there are other symptoms to come back. Otherwise, get in touch with her doctor on Monday. The glands are still swollen, so heaven knows what's going on. The ER doctor couldn't find any reason for it and said glands sometimes swell for reasons unknown. Very reassuring, but as long as she seems to feel okay otherwise, I guess we won't worry right now. We're going to friends for dinner this afternoon. Hope you have a good day. Love, Kay

NOTE: The swollen glands incident was an instance of the frustrations of dealing with doctors. The ER doctor clearly had no idea what was causing it. When I spoke on the phone to her oncologist two days later, she wasn't phased at all—the swollen glands were a typical manifestation of the steroid Stel was taking. Nothing to worry about and nothing to be done about it.

Section 2. The Next Six Months

Thu Jan 06 2000 8:42 AM

Dear Mary, Stel has continued to have problems for the past few weeks—mainly balance and walking (and not being able to do much for herself). Monday a week ago (12/27), she was so bad that I couldn't deal with her by myself at home. She actually fell the night before and I had a hell of a time getting her off the floor. The doctor put her in the hospital and upped the Decadron dose. Her balance and walking improved significantly in a few days. By New Year's Eve she was doing well enough that I was able to persuade the doctor to let her out of the hospital so I could take her to a small hotel in Bethesda, where we had a pleasant New Year's Eve and Day. It was a welcome respite and felt like a mini-vacation. We checked her back into the hospital on Sunday evening (the doctor and I wanted to keep her there until the social workers had set up all home therapy and assistance possible). By Tuesday, she was doing so well—she improved a lot cognitively as well—and the social workers had gotten everything in process, so we came home. Almost as soon as we walked in the door, Stel started having walking problems she didn't seem to have at the hospital—very frustrating. She did somewhat better yesterday, and we had a wheelchair delivered, which helps a lot. The main problem with the wheelchair is that there are ten steps up to our apartment and there's no disabled access or possibility of it without extensive changes. Stel hasn't had much trouble going up the stairs but she has a lot of trouble now going down—it frightens her. I'm desperately trying to find another apartment, or even a condo to buy, that doesn't have the stair problem and also is more compact than our present apartment, which has a long hallway to the bedroom. Of course, we live in the most ridiculously expensive part of the D.C. area and prices for anything approaching what we now have are ludicrous. But I've got to do something soon if I'm going to make life easier for both of us. Just what I need—another challenge to deal with.

Stel started CCNU while she was in the hospital. I had planned to give it to her at home but since she was in the hospital, they gave it to her there. So far no side effects that we know of. She'll get her white cell count tested next week. Hopefully, it will be okay since I've been giving her supplements for some time to boost her immune system, as well as putting chlorophyll in her water. (Friends who saw Stel in the hospital for the first time since last year were amazed to see how well she looks and relates. They didn't think she looked sick at all, despite her moon face and her still very sparse hair. I took a great picture of her about a month ago in a jaunty hat I bought her and you'd never have a clue she's ill from looking at it. That's one of the many pernicious things about these beasts in the head.)

Stel's MRI last week as a follow-up to the SR procedure shows no new growth, which is what the doctor in Chicago said they would be looking for on the first scan. In a month, she'll get another MRI to see how the CCNU is doing. From that Friedman will decide whether to do another round or switch to something else. (We liked Dr. Friedman a lot when we met him. He's very informal and down to earth and made us feel that he would stay on top of the treatment. Also, the facility at Duke is certainly more pleasant to go to than Hopkins. We both came away from Hopkins feeling depressed. Of course, Duke is a lot further away. Our local oncologist liked talking to Friedman, too. She said he "wasn't full of himself." I'm glad they get along well, so I think there will be good cooperation between them. If Stel's up to it in a few weeks, Friedman said he'd like to see her again, but we'll see how it goes. We actually enjoyed the trip down there because the weather was so nice and we broke the drive up into 2- or 3-hour segments, so it took 3 nights to go and come back. Despite seeing doctors, it also seemed like a vacation. I hope if we go back I can get someone to go with us so I'll have some help. It would make it easier.)

As I said, Stel has improved cognitively in the last several days. I'm hoping she'll continue to come out of the fog she's in—she's getting home speech therapy, as well as PT and OT, and we'll have a home aide for personal care. I'm going to pay extra for some additional hours of home assistance a couple of times a week to give me a break and maybe make it possible for me to do a little part-time work at home, if things stay halfway stable for a while.

Stel is still laughing at herself; still a sweetheart, loved by all nurses and attendants because she's so good-natured and kind to them. She's remarkable, as I've always known. Here's to a better New Year for all of us. All the best, Kay

Mon Jan 17 2000 8:40 AM

Dear Dr. Friedman, I wondered whether you can shed any light on what's happening with Stel. Her MRI taken on 12/30 as a follow-up to the radiosurgery procedure showed no significant change from the one taken on 12/1, the day before the procedure. She took CCNU—220mg—on December 28th. She was in the hospital from 12/27 to 1/3 primarily because her balance and walking were so bad that I couldn't deal with her by myself at home and her oncologist wanted to get the hospital social workers to help get as much home care set up as possible. Stel's Decadron dose was increased from 12 mg to 20 while she was in the hospital. By the time she came home, her balance was better and she was walking, with assistance, fairly well. Almost as soon as she got home, though, she started having balance and walking problems again (no change at that point in steroid dose.) In the last two weeks, she's been very erratic. Some days I think she's improving greatly and other days, like yesterday, she seems unable to hold her balance at all. (She's having home physical therapy. I asked the therapist if he thought the chemo might be causing any of these problems and he seemed to think it was possible that she might feel weaker as a result of the workings of the drug. However, I don't understand why it would be that way one day, or one part of one day, but not another.) Also, cognitively, she goes from being very unresponsive and just wanting to stare at the TV all day, even needing help with eating sometimes, to being much more "with it" and able to engage in limited conversation. For several days last weekend and early in the week, she was just gone; then she suddenly was much more animated and was that way for about three days. Then yesterday, she was once again very unresponsive and lethargic.

I just wondered whether you might have any thoughts about what's going on. We saw Dr. Raj last Tuesday, when Stel was in a nonresponsive state. Her only thought was to increase the steroid dose, from 12 back up to 20 for a couple of days. For the last three days, Stel's been on 16. I haven't really been able to see much difference in the effect on her walking/balance. I know these tumors and treatments have unpredictable courses and there may not be a good explanation for this, but it just seems, given the MRI, that she shouldn't be having this much trouble. I'd appreciate any thoughts you have. Thanks, Kay Loveland

Tue Jan 18 2000 1:22 AM

Dear Mary, Things aren't good, I'm afraid. Stel's situation is very erratic. Her walking and balance are not good but some days they appear to be getting better and then the next day they're worse and she seems unable to take any steps at all. Even more troubling to me, she's often really out of it these days. She'll be okay, engaging with me and then zonk out and be almost completely unresponsive. Today was one of those days and it's really hard to take. Our local oncologist whom we saw this week didn't have any good explanations for it; she just upped the steroid dose, but I can't see that it has any significant effect on these problems. Yesterday I e-mailed Dr. Friedman to ask for his thoughts. It's very depressing and discouraging. On top of everything else, Stel is usually unable to avoid wetting herself at night and she's had a few problems during the day as well. The only thing that keeps me from freaking out completely is that Jeanne Wallace said she's seen BT patients in worse shape who have recovered substantially. I'm hoping that will be the case with Stel. Right now there's just no apparent physical reason why she should be doing worse. Her MRI on the 30th showed no new growth or swelling.

I'm facing the same difficulty with Stel that you have with your sister—holding her up, getting her up, keeping her from falling. I'm stronger than I ever could have imagined and have a good back, apparently, but my body is really feeling the strain these days. Fortunately, Stel and I are about the same weight, but to really handle her without a lot of stress, I need more muscles. The doctor upset me earlier in the week by saying Stel should go to a long-term care facility because it was too much for me. I told her this just isn't an answer, so I'm now really trying to line up respite care. I should have more I can tell you about this in a couple of days. For the moment, we have a home aide coming in three times a week just for an hour or so to help Stel get cleaned up. Insurance is paying for this. But, of course, I need more. A social worker gave me numbers for some places and people to call and I'm going to do that tomorrow or Wednesday. I'll let you know what I find out. Please let me know what you discover as well.

As for the chemo (CCNU), so far Stel's not having the side effects they said she might—nausea or low white blood count, but her appetite has dropped off despite the steroids, which can be a side effect. And I'm wondering if the drugs aren't having more impact on her behavior than we might think. I just pray the next scan will show signs of positive effect.

A major problem for us now is the steps leading up to the landing of our apartment. It's just not doable any more for Stel and we're really trapped here now. I have managed to get her out to a doctor's appointment and to the ER the other night (for swollen ankles), but it's less and less feasible. I don't know how I'm going to manage to get her to the MRI in a couple of weeks. (A social worker told me she didn't know of a service that would help me get Stel out of the apartment and take her to her appointment, but I can't believe there isn't one. Somehow I've got to find it.) Because of this, I've been frantically looking for another place to live. I think I've found another apartment in Bethesda but, of course, I'm going to have to pay almost twice as much rent as I'm paying now. I guess I'll try to get moved in mid- to late-February. I'm relying on the assurance of friends that they'll pitch in because there's no way I can do this without a lot of help. That's it for now. Best wishes, Kay

Tue Jan 18 2000 5:16 PM

To Kay Loveland. This up and down is not unusual—work with your home MD to try and continue giving her the chance to respond. Henry [Friedman]

Thu Jan 20 2000 7:17 AM
Subject: HELP:STEL CAN'T DO ANYTHING FOR HERSELF

Dear friends [BT List], I haven't posted in quite a while because the last several weeks have been frantic and exhausting and I haven't even had time to read messages on the digest I've been on, let alone write a message. Any light, support, help, words of wisdom any of you can shed on any aspect of what follows would be deeply appreciated. (Sorry, this is a lot longer than I intended.)

My partner Stel had sterotactic radiosurgery at CINN on December 2nd and she hasn't been the same since. Before we had the procedure, we spoke to Dr. Helenowski, who performed it, several times and asked every question we could think of about risks and benefits. Stel made a decision to do it after we'd had many discussions with local docs and friends and talked about it ourselves more than once. (Her first follow-up MRI on 12/30 appears to indicate that the radiosurgery did stop the tumor in its tracks for the moment.)

When I saw her for a couple of hours the after the procedure, she seemed herself and I was relieved. But the next morning when I came in to get her ready to check out of the hospital, she had bad twitches in both arms and was very much out of it. And she couldn't walk. After an EEG and CT scan, the doctors decided she'd had a seizure. The next morning, fortunately, we were able to check her out of the hospital and fly home. She was able to climb the ten steps up to the landing of our apartment with support from me and a friend. But it soon became apparent that she just wasn't functioning as she had been. She was taking an inordinately long time sitting on the toilet and washing her hands (running the water) afterwards, which, it became clear, she knew was absurd (she laughed about it). And she was no longer able to initiate anything for herself. Basically, she usually just wants to sit in front of the TV and watch whatever is on. She doesn't attempt to change channels; she can't dial a phone number and when she talks on the phone, she doesn't hang up after the other person does; she just sits and listens, and sometimes talks, to a dead phone. At first I had to feed her to get her to eat and sometimes I still have to do that. If she eats herself, she pushes a lot of her food off her plate and may spend well over an hour eating. I can't entrust her pill taking to her any more because she'll just sit and stare at the pills. She's usually unable to finish her sentences and will end them with whatever she's seeing on TV. In particular, she never seems to be able to tell me how to help her if she needs something; she'll just repeat back to me my questions. She can't write her name now, or anything else. If she starts it okay, it ends in squiggles. (Stel was having out-patient PT, OT, and speech therapy before we went to Chicago but her functioning level was so much lower when we returned that the therapists recommended she go back to home therapy.) She wets herself every night now and on occasion has done so during the day, as well as not making it to the toilet for bowel movements on 2-3 occasions (she doesn't tell me when she needs to go—although she did say yesterday that she needed to "change, change" and I decided that meant go to the bathroom and got her there in time for a bowel movement).

Her balance has been very bad for several weeks and she's often unable to take any steps at all. She's now in a wheelchair all the time. Going down the steps from our apartment became exceedingly difficult after we came back from Chicago because she was so frightened to do it, and it's become impossible now without considerable additional help. This is a BIG problem since I haven't found any service that is willing to get her out of the apartment and into a vehicle to take her to appointments or anything else. (I'm frantically trying to get us moved in the next month or so.) Because of her walking problems, which have made it very hard for me to deal with her alone at home, she's been in and out of the hospital twice since we came back from Chicago. I'm trying to get substantial respite care set up at home. IF ANYONE HAS ANY SUGGESTIONS ABOUT WHERE TO FIND HELP WITH TRANSPORTATION OR RESPITE CARE IN THE WASHINGTON, D.C. AREA, PLEASE ADVISE.

Among the many distressing and frustrating things I'm encountering is that at times Stel is much more "with it." After the first week at home from Chicago, she seemed to improve somewhat and was able to communicate a little better and answer questions. She was responsive to the speech therapist's requests in her first couple of visits. She became more animated. She tried in small ways to do a few things for herself, although she still couldn't initiate much, but she was much more herself. However, in the last couple of weeks, she'll often "zone out" and be almost completely unresponsive, as she was during the first week home. Last week she had about three days when she was "with it." Yesterday morning when she woke up, she was much more herself—talking, making little jokes; then, after I spent an hour struggling to get her cleaned up (the home aide didn't show up as scheduled), which took a great deal of energy on both our parts, she was zoned out again and stayed that way all day. I can't tell whether it's just that she gets so fatigued she can't make the effort to interact; that's what it seemed like yesterday.

I don't mean to say that none of these problems existed before the radiosurgery. She was having balance and walking difficulties for about three weeks before. She was much less able to initiate things since her second surgery in August, but she was able to do more than she can now—in fact, she was beginning to cook a few things (which she loves to do) before. Now that's impossible. I have a hard time getting her to tell me how to cook favorite recipes; she just can't do the sequencing. She also could attempt to dress herself—albeit very slowly—before; now she doesn't even try. She took more interest in projects and TV programs, movies, politics, etc. before and usually had opinions to express (Stel was always a person of strong opinions); since radiosurgery she seems pretty much a blank slate. Before the procedure, she was having some memory problems, some aphasia problems, some handwriting problems, some incontinence at night, but it all seems to be greatly exacerbated now. I don't know that a direct causal link can be made, but it seems likely to me that the procedure did inflict some of this damage.

I have to throw into the mix here that on 12/28 Stel had her first round of CCNU, and I'm wondering whether the workings of the drug may be causing some of her problems, particularly the zoning out and in. Could that be a result of fatigue from the chemo? Or something else?

Dr. Friedman at Duke says these ups and downs are not that unusual and we just have to give Stel time to respond to the treatments. Jeanne Wallace says she's seen BT patients in worse shape who've recovered a lot of their functioning. I'd really appreciate any advice anyone has who's been through any of this, or who has medical knowledge about these things. I fear that I've lost my beloved sidekick, partner, and pal of thirty-plus years, that she'll never really be herself again, and maybe if she hadn't had radiosurgery this wouldn't have happened, at least for a while longer. Thanks for taking time to read this and respond. Kay Loveland

Thu Jan 20 2000 4:24 PM

Dear Sharon, Providing home health care so people can stay at home only makes good sense, doesn't it? Unfortunately, there's not much of it here. There is a volunteer group, Hospice Caring, that is non-medical and doesn't require a terminal declaration in order to provide respite care. Someone is coming to talk to us on Monday. I think they may be able to fill the bill for us now. Also, there's a group for lesbians with cancer in D.C. that has been providing different kinds of help for the past several months and they're trying to get some people who can do some respite for me. If I can get this resolved and get us out of this apartment soon, maybe I can get things a little more under control for the moment. Of course, that depends completely on whether Stel's MRI next week remains stable or better. Otherwise, we return to the mad scramble.

As for her immune system, I've been giving her every healthy thing I can lay my hands on since May. And since October we've been working with a nutritionist who works with brain tumor patients and has had some success, so far as one can tell. I hope Stel's immune system isn't devastated. Her blood test ten days ago for white count and platelets was, according to the doctor, "perfect." Will know better next week when she gets another test after the chemo has had four weeks to work. But none of these good things, including the "good" MRI of last month seem to have any effect on how she's functioning. God, this disease is a horror! Thanks for the hugs and good wishes. We'll keep them close to our hearts. Kay

Thu Jan 20 2000 7:47 PM

Dear Mary, Thanks for your message. Did the nurse say why it's common for patients to get worse even when their MRIs show no change, and did she say whether they can get better? Dr. Helenowski's office called from Chicago to say that he looked at the 12/30 MRI and found that the tumor was "stable if not slightly smaller."

I've been calling to try to solve the problem of getting Stel out of the apartment to appointments. You'd think it had never happened in the history of the universe that someone living in an apartment with stairs becomes too ill to be able to deal with them and needs help. None of the organizations I called will take on getting her down the stairs. Finally, a woman who is disabled whom I know slightly directed me to a driver for a cab company (they have wheelchair vans). He does carry people in and out of buildings, etc. I'll have to call him and see if he can help us. Warm wishes for now, Kay

Sat Jan 22 2000 8:26 AM

Dear Sharon, Your message of love and caring means a lot. And no, I don't think you've gone around the bend. I have long thought it didn't make sense that our spirits, souls, whatever one wants to call it, are snuffed out when our physical selves are. I suspect there's something more there, and the (Buddhist?) idea of a cosmic energy force that we're all a part of seems a possibility. I don't have the answers, but I, like you, doubt that our spirits are constrained by our bodies. Certainly, Stel's soul is so great that I believe it must transcend the constraints of her physical self. Keep your good thoughts coming, Kay

Sun Jan 23 2000 8:37 AM

Dear George, If you have the time to do any research on books or articles about brain regeneration and find anything that would be understandable to the lay person, please let me know. I'd like to find out whatever I can about what the possibilities are that Stel may, can, could regain some of her cognitive abilities if the tumor is kept in check. Thanks, Kay

Sun Jan 23 2000 9:05 AM

Dear Karla, Stel and I appreciate your lovely note of caring and concern. Stel says to tell you that you are her adopted niece. Certainly, she's had no such expressions of caring from her own nieces and nephews (one wonders how Stel could have come out of that family).

So far the news is pretty depressing. Stel's really unable to do anything for herself and has a lot of memory and concentration problems. I took heart this morning, though, in a message I saw about a woman who has had at least six brain operations over the past several years and many other kinds of treatments. Most recently, she had surgery in September and has been in hospital and rehab ever since. She was unable to walk for three months and had severe disorientation and other cognitive problems. The message said that she is now walking with a walker and her mind is back to normal. I'm hoping beyond hope that I'll be able to send a similar message in a few months. If the tumor shrinks, that will give Stel a good shot at some recovery. It's at least stopped in its tracks for the moment, according to the last MRI. Pray that the next one at the end of this week will give us some good news that we can build on.

A major problem now is that I can't get Stel up and down the stairs by myself safely, so we're really stuck in the apartment. It's a huge undertaking to find assistance to get her to appointments. Because of this, we've got to move and I've put in an application on an apartment in an elevator building. If I can line up a brigade to help pack and move, I think we'll probably do it in mid to late February. It's an overwhelming thought but has to be done. Also, I'm struggling to get as much respite care as I can to help me at home. When Stel is as non-functional as she is now, I end up doing a lot of heavy lifting and, while I'm very strong and have a good back, I'm feeling the strain. It's just too much to do everything and, unfortunately, we've got no one here who can take a substantial part of the load on a regular basis. I hope by the end of the week to have a schedule of daily help set up. We're also now getting regular delivery of meals three times a week from a cancer support group and the Unitarian Church. Every little bit helps a lot. That's the story for now. Hugs to both of you. Love, Kay

Tue Jan 25 2000 3:34 AM
Subject: HELP

Friends, Stel and I have just come back from a third visit to the emergency room in the past month—this time for abdominal pains; previously for swollen ankles and swollen glands. Once again they found nothing significant and sent her home with medicine for constipation. We are now waiting for it to work. Getting to and from the emergency room, or anywhere else these days, is impossible for the two of us to manage alone. Today a 911 crew took her there because she was crying out in such pain. I had gone out for an hour to run some errands and had a volunteer staying with Stel. When I came back, the ambulance was in the parking lot and I couldn't believe my eyes. Just two hours before, Faith and I had managed with considerable effort to get Stel to the bathroom and to bed for a nap and when I left, she was resting peacefully.

I can't begin to recount for you how our days are filled. There's rarely a day that goes by that doesn't have a surprise—usually not a pleasant one—and they are most often frantic with putting out fires and calling doctors, therapists, social workers, and following leads about treatments, respite care, transportation, apartments, etc. This past week, I've worked on lining up as much respite care as I can in the short term—there may be some longer-term possibilities when I can get applications filled out and submitted. I've also found an apartment and tentatively talked to movers about moving around February 21st. I'll have the date and mover nailed down in a couple of days. Also, with the help of people from the Unitarian Church and others, meals are now coming on schedule three times a week. This is all helpful, but given the overwhelming nature of the situation, I need even more.

I'm almost as bad as Stel in asking for help for myself, but when it comes to her, I can do it. As most of you know, right now Stel isn't functioning well at all. Her balance and walking are extremely bad sometimes, like today, and somewhat better other times—I've stopped thinking those times indicate she's beginning to improve. The same is true with her ability to interact and respond. There are times when she's much more herself and, unfortunately, more times lately when she's pretty much out of it. Since so far as we know right now the tumor is at least stable, if not shrinking, and there hasn't been any substantial increase in swelling, the doctors have no good explanations for why she's not doing better, except to say brain tumor patients have these ups and downs and, hopefully, she'll regain some of her ability to function if and when the treatments are effective. There are quite a few inspiring stories of people in the same or worse shape who have come back a long way. I've contacted a neuro-psychologist who is actually going to make a house call on Wednesday morning, given the difficulty I have in getting Stel out of the apartment. She, working with a neuro-psychiatrist, may be able to offer some new options for helping Stel cognitively. I'm hoping so, at least. I'm also thinking, as of today, that Stel probably needs more intensive physical, occupational, and cognitive therapy than she's getting at home if she's going to regain any of her strength and I've got to find an acceptable place for her to get that kind of help soon. Not an easy task.

The long and short of it is, we need all the help we can get at the moment. I know you're all very busy people and, like Stel, hate to impose upon your time and subject you to a depressing situation, but the circumstances give me no options. I appreciate deeply everything you've already done. I hope you'll be able to find time to do more for Stel in coming weeks. As some of you know, I'm going to be needing a lot of help in packing and unpacking in the days before and after our move. I'll appreciate whatever you can do in that regard. Additional help with cooking and meals would also be gratefully accepted. And whenever you can find time to spend with Stel, I hope you will. Our new apartment will be more central and, hopefully, will make it easier to stop by from time to time. If visits aren't always possible, phone calls (or e-mails) every few days to check in and say hello also lift the spirits. (If Stel's not up to talking much, as she often isn't these days, I know seeing and hearing from you still brightens the day, for her and me). Right now, being pretty much trapped in the apartment as we are, visits and phone calls are especially welcome.

What more can I say? God knows I wish I didn't have to ask you for help. God knows I wish Stel and I could be planning our long-anticipated trip to the Baltic. God knows I wish we could go back to last year at this time and erase everything that's happened since April 21st. Since I can't, all I can say is HELP. Many thanks, Kay

Thu Jan 27 2000 7:54 AM

Dear Donna, Thanks so much for your message. I had surmised that Anne was your partner and I'm glad to be able to communicate with you directly. This is all so painful, and now I fear I won't even have the comfort of having Stel at home with me to care for, hug, kiss, and whisper sweet nothings to. If she can't hold her balance or help me move her around at little, I'm unable to handle her by myself. I had begun to line up some good respite care this week and thought I would be able to get us in a situation where it would be doable at home, but then I came to the very reluctant decision that if she doesn't get more intensive rehab, she's got no possibility of getting stronger. So I've got to find a place for her to be nearby for a few weeks. I pray that she will be able to get back to a point where it's easier to have her with me.

I can't bear the thought of us not being together for the rest of our lives—however long or short that may be. I already feel like the person I've been with all these years is mostly gone, and it's a very lonely feeling, but there are flashes of her old self and there is still her wonderful warm, soft body and skin and lips, and her beautiful eyes and it means a lot just to hold her. I've got to hold on to that for as long as possible. I know it must be terribly difficult for you to be without Anne. I can't even envision a future without Stella, my sidekick, partner, pal, lover for more than thirty years. Kay

Fri Jan 28 2000 8:32 AM

Dear Charles, It's good to hear from you. Needless to say, my heart is shattered at what has happened. Stel has never had an easy time and now to face this horror is really too much to bear, but we have no choice. I wouldn't believe in fate, except

I've lived it for thirty years with Stella. (At every step of the way since April, I've thought surely it can't be the worst news; surely Stel will get some break. At every step it's been worse than I could imagine. She has the worst type of tumor, in a very bad location, and now she's suffering from just about every deficit possible. The only solace is that she's had no significant pain so far.) It's been a nightmare since April.

I'm really doing everything for her now. I suspect the powerful drugs she's taking may be causing some of her lethargy problems these days. Stel never took drugs and was always very sensitive to them; now she's taking steroids, anti-seizure medications, and chemo drugs. I've just reluctantly decided that I've got to get her back into intensive rehab if she's going to be functional enough to help me move her around. So I hope I can find an acceptable place close to where we live for her to spend a few weeks, and I pray in a few weeks she'll be in good enough shape that I can have her at home with respite help. I know of people in as bad or worse shape than Stel who have regained a lot of functionality. She's been remarkable up until now and I hope that will continue.

Stel's also been remarkable in her ability to see the absurdity and irony of the awful situation she's in. And she's a sweetheart in every way. I love her so much and my heart aches so much for her. The situation for us is a disaster on every level. I haven't been able to work since August. Fortunately, I've been the recipient of a lot of donated federal leave that I've been able to stretch out over these months so I could get half a pay check. I had hoped to be able to do some part-time work at home if and when Stel were stable enough and I got some help, but it doesn't appear that situation will come about for another month or two at the earliest. On top of everything else, I've got to move us because the apartment we're in has steps that have become a major obstacle. I've enlisted a brigade of people to help me move to a smaller place. At least once Stel is a little stronger, I can bring her home to a building that doesn't pose an obstacle course just getting into and out of it.

God knows I wish you and others we know were nearby. Unfortunately, all of our oldest and closest friends are in far-flung places. We're really stranded here. We do have some good friends who have been very supportive, and I have a connection with a Unitarian Church that has helped a lot; there's also a lesbian group that's offering assistance. But none of it is as sustained as the help we would get from friends who are in other places. Of course, our families are of little help, financially or otherwise. My sister came up in July for a week and was very helpful, and she'll come back sometime soon. Must run. Thanks for writing. Love, Kay

Mon Jan 31 2000 8:27 AM

Dear Mary, As usual, things haven't gone smoothly here these past days. I was beginning to line up some respite help—not as much as I had hoped since most of the volunteers are older and aren't trained in transfers, so they can't give me the basic help I need in moving Stel around. Also, getting help in the morning and during the day isn't as easy as getting it in the evening. But a young woman has come over a couple of mornings and been a great help in getting Stel up. But I've decided I have to get Stel into a somewhat intensive rehab program if she's going to regain any strength. Although she's a bit stronger and her balance is a little better these last couple of days, she's nowhere near where she needs to be for me to be able to deal with her here. I think she'll be transferred to the hospital today and then I've got to find an acceptable rehab place in the Bethesda area. I hate to put her in a facility and hope to hell I can get her a private room. Those semi-privates are the pits, and so depressing. I hope, too, that after maybe three weeks, she'll be improved enough I can bring her home to the new apartment and have enough help lined up to make things work better than they have the last several weeks. It's just got to get better, as I keep telling Stel. Let me know how things are going with your sister. Kay

Wed Feb 02 2000 8:00 AM

Dear Peter, I'd appreciate it if you (or someone in Sweden) could find out more about what's happening in Lund regarding brain tumors. (See the attached message.) I know I'll never have time to contact the doctors myself.

Stel is doing much better cognitively. This started day before yesterday—she was suddenly carrying on conversations with me, and she said, "I think I'm coming back." She's back in the hospital as of yesterday (and taking a little Ritalin to help even more with cognition—it seems to be working) while we decide on where she will go for rehab. I'm so happy to have her talking to me again. It's a great relief. Also, she had an MRI yesterday. We haven't gotten the official read on it yet, but I looked at it with the oncologist last night and it appears to us that there is some improvement. So far I've been right when I look at these godawful scans. Kay

Thu Feb 03 2000 8:10 AM

Dear Peter, The attached message I just got appears to give pretty inclusive information about what's happening in Lund [an immunization trial for people already diagnosed with a BT that won't yield results for at least two years]. I don't know that there's anything more you or your contacts in Sweden could get right now. This treatment in Lund (and apparently at Duke) sounds like something to hope for, but two years or more is an eternity in the world Stel and I are now living in.

Stel continues to do well—lively and talkative. The radiologist says the MRI shows a stable and perhaps slightly smaller tumor. I think it's definitely a little smaller. It certainly looks better than it did two months ago when we went to Chicago. She will probably be transferred to a rehab facility in Chevy Chase, about ten minutes from our place, sometime today. Warm regards, Kay

Thu Feb 03 2000 8:25 AM

Dear Cathy, Sorry I haven't gotten back to you. Stel will probably be moving to a rehab facility sometime today. She continues to do well with communication—lively and talkative—and that's wonderful. Based on a good MRI last week, her oncologists will decide, probably today, about a second round of chemo for her. She's ready to get to rehab and begin working to regain her strength. I'll let you know the phone number there when I get it. Kay

Fri Feb 04 2000 11:41 PM

Dear friends [on BT List], For almost two months my partner Stel has been very unresponsive and uncommunicative, seemingly out in space much of the time and unable to function in any way. Suddenly, last Monday she began to "come back," as she said, and actually began to have conversations with me. That very night, her oncologist put her on a small dose of Ritalin (5 mg a day), which we had discussed earlier, and for the past three days she's been even more lively, much more her old self. The neurologist was worried about seizures and did an EEG, which showed nothing. He's watching her seizure medicine levels (Tegretol and Depakote) closely. So far, no problems, and Stel has even begun to initiate a few things. It gives us both a lot of hope. Kay

Sat Feb 19 2000 12:11 AM

Dear Robin, Hope things are going okay with you. I'm in the midst of getting us packed for moving on the 22nd. A lot of good samaritans are doing the packing; I'm directing. Stel has been in rehab two weeks and has made some progress in her balance and walking ability; cognitively, she's more herself. But she's got a long way to go to regain any significant functioning. I think I've got to look for therapists who deal with brain injuries/tumors more frequently who know how to deal with the special problems they entail. These pretty much want to write her off because of her "poor prognosis." That's just not going to happen. I hope to keep her there another couple of weeks until I get moved in and somewhat organized and, hopefully, line up some good respite care to help me. Then I want to look further for the right people to help her make further progress.

She took her second round of CCNU last week and will have another MRI in early March. Then, Henry Friedman wants to give her a couple of rounds of Temodar, then maybe CPT-11. She seems to be doing okay with this aspect of things, but all of her systems have just gone haywire for who knows what reason. Let me hear from you. Best, Kay

Mon Feb 21 2000 8:14 AM

Dear Ann, How am I doing? Overwhelmed is the word. I'm moving tomorrow and have been spending every spare minute organizing things for the good samaritans who have been packing for me. Everything's just about done. We're moving to an apartment in an elevator building so we don't have to contend with the few steps up to the landing here. I'm paying $1,800 a month for the privilege, but there just isn't any choice. Stel has been in a rehab facility for the last two-plus weeks. She's gotten stronger, her balance is better, but she still has a lot of problems. I'm hoping to take her home in another week or two, with some help at home, but I've got to keep looking for the right therapists to help her. She needs people who work with these problems all the time and she hasn't got them now. Anyway, I'm there most of the day and at home early mornings and late evenings organizing and packing. I'll be glad to get the move out of the way. Thanks for keeping in touch. Love, Kay

Sat Feb 26 2000 8:55 AM

Dear Moira, Stel has gotten stronger in the rehab place but still can't walk very well. The National Rehab Hospital has said they will take her now in their brain injury unit for acute rehab, but we're waiting to see whether Blue Cross approves it. Even if they don't, I'll probably pay for it myself to give her a chance to have some significant treatment there. I think it's the best hope she has for more significant progress. She's better cognitively than she was for a while, but still not the old Stel. She's taken her second round of chemo. The last MRI scan looked stable, if not slightly smaller. She'll have another one in a couple of weeks and, hopefully, it'll show a decrease if the chemo is being effective. Hope all is well with you. Kay

Mon Feb 28, 2000 10:58 PM

Dear Peter, I don't have time now to tell you all that has transpired at the rehab place the past three weeks. Suffice to say that Stel got some good therapy but not as much as she should have. She's gotten stronger—better balance and getting up and down. Walking remains very erratic. Cognitively she's been pretty bright but still has many problems. Because of the mess the therapists have made out of things, today is the last day Blue Cross is paying for the rehab place. I was planning to bring her home to the new apartment tomorrow, but got word Friday that the brain injury unit of the National Rehab Hospital in D.C. would be willing to take her for intensive therapy for a week or two. It's the best place in this area for therapy with people who really know how to deal with the problems Stel has and would be the best chance she'd have right now to make significant progress, if possible. However, Blue Cross is saying they won't pay for it. I'm determined to have her there for at least a week and will pay the $1,000 a day if I have to. The oncologist is trying to get the insurance company to change its mind. If so, Stel will be transferred there. If not, I may try to get the hospital to agree to let her come next Monday so she can get a full week of intensive therapy rather than going mid-week when she'll be there on the weekend without a full therapy schedule. If they agree to that, I'll bring her home for the intervening period.

I had hoped she'd be able to keep tapering down the steroid she's been on because of the bad side effects it can have and it had gone down some, but unfortunately she had a seizure this morning and the doctor has raised it again.

I hope with all my heart that Stel gets strong enough to make the trip to Sweden in June. It's impossible to know now; everything is so unpredictable. I know that if she is able to go, I'm going to have to have someone accompany us because I can't handle it all by myself.

I'll let you know where we are as soon as I know. The move to the new apartment went pretty smoothly, with a lot of help from friends, and I'm at least able to function in the place right now, even though there are still boxes to unpack, organizing to do to get everything in place. That's it for now. Love, Kay

Wed Mar 01 2000 11:51 PM

Dear Barbara, We're moved in. I'd love to say come by next Wednesday, but we won't be here then. Stel just came from rehab today and will be here through the weekend. Then on Monday morning I'm taking her to the National Rehab Hospital in D.C., where she'll get intensive therapy for at least a week. Blue Cross has said they won't pay for it (because the therapists in the last place didn't know how to deal with Stel and made them think she can't benefit from more intensive therapy), so I'm going to be forking over the cash to give her that chance. I just think she deserves to have the best people around here who deal with these kinds of problems all the time work with her, since they've said they'd be willing to give it a shot. The insurance company isn't going to deny that to her. I'm not a rich person—getting poorer all the time—but her life and the quality of it is worth far more to me than a few thousand dollars. She did get stronger with the less-than-optimum therapy she had and I pray she'll make greater gains with better people. She'll also get a complete cognitive evaluation, which I'd like to have.

Please plan to come by on another Wednesday. I'd like to try to make the BT meeting on the 3rd Thursday, but it will depend on whether Stel's home (which she should be) and whether I've got someone to stay with her. We'll see. Hope things are all right for you and Mark and the kids. It's good to have Stel at home, where I can crawl into bed next to her, which is what I'm about to do. Take care, Kay

Fri Mar 03 2000 12:05 AM

Dr. Friedman, Stel took her second round of CCNU on February 9th. She's tolerating it well, but continues to have a lot of difficulty moving her legs and functioning in other ways. She's been in in-patient rehab for three weeks and has gotten stronger, but the therapists really didn't know what to do with her (they're used to old people with broken hips, etc.) and didn't give her as much help as they could, I believe. Next week I'm taking her to the National Rehab Hospital in D.C. They've said they'd take her on a trial basis for a week or two. Even though Blue Cross is refusing to pay, Stel wants this chance to have people who know more about her situation work with her and I want her to have it, too. It's her best shot for the moment. It's just so frustrating that the MRIs look pretty good and she's doing okay on the chemo, yet she's not functioning well. Kay Loveland

Mon Mar 06 2000 11:35 PM

Dear Ann, The move went pretty well and the new apartment is okay. Paying the rent is a traumatic experience, however. Stel left the rehab facility last Wednesday and came home through the weekend. Today I took her to the Brain Injury Unit of the National Rehab Hospital for intensive therapy. I hope she can make some significant progress in about a week. Blue Cross has refused to pay for it, contending she won't benefit from it—even though NRH felt she might. I'm going to appeal the decision and hopefully they'll ultimately have to pay up. In addition to therapy, they'll take a comprehensive look at the hodge podge of medications she's on and maybe come up with a regimen that is less likely to zonk her out much of the time.

As for my job, I had hoped since November to be able to do some part-time work at home, but that hasn't ever been feasible. IF Stel's medical condition stays stable during the next few months and she's tolerating the chemo pretty well, and IF I can knit together enough volunteer and paid help at home to free up some hours, I'll try to do some work mostly at home. The office has asked me to update a manual that I edited a few years ago. It's tedious work but can be done away from the office and with no firm deadline, so I'm hoping I'll be able to do that. If I can't, I'll continue to get half a pay check from donated leave into May and then I can use some sick leave under the Family Friendly Leave Act. When those options run out, I'll have to take an official leave of absence. At this point, I have no idea what tomorrow will bring, let alone a month or two down the road. It's just a frantic scramble nearly all the time. Thanks for your concern. Kay

Fri Mar 10 2000 11:40 PM

Dear Mary, Stel has been at the National Rehab Hospital this week, and she's had a remarkable couple of days yesterday and today. She's much more alert on a constant basis, much more communicative, and has really tried to do what the therapists wanted and, in most cases, has been able to do it. She surpassed even their expectations because they, too, saw the diagnosis and wanted to tell me that she probably wasn't going to get any better. I'd keep her there another week now, but we're making some adjustments in her anti-seizure meds (phasing down Depakote because I think it's been a factor in her lack of responsiveness over these months and the doctors agreed it could be) and need to see what that does for her. Also, she's got to take another round of chemo in the next week or so and I don't know how that will affect her. She'll have at-home PT/OT and then in 2-3 weeks we'll see whether it makes sense for her to go back to the hospital for another round of intensive therapy. In the meantime, I'll appeal Blue Cross's refusal to pay, accompanied by reports from NRH therapists and, hopefully, get them to pay up. I have so much time to do that, of course.

At any rate, I'm very happy tonight because of the improvements I've seen in Stel for the last two days. She's been remarkable, so determined and yet so sweet at the same time. I just pray the improvement lasts and, perhaps, means the chemo is working. She still has a long way to go; she can't walk much at all and can't do anything without a lot of help, but maybe she's on the road back to better times. She'll have another MRI on Sunday. If things look pretty good, Friedman probably will switch to Temodar. I'm nervous about it because I don't know whether she'll tolerate it as well as the CCNU and, of course, if it looks like the CCNU is having a good effect, it'll be a gamble as to whether Temodar will do as well. But I also agree with him and others that it makes sense to attack these beasts with more than one chemo at a time to try to avoid its building up chemo resistance.

Better get to bed. I'm bringing Stel home tomorrow. Still haven't got enough home care lined up but hope to get that in place within 2-3 weeks. All good wishes, Kay

Sat Mar 11 2000 7:53 AM

Dear Carole, Stel had another remarkable day yesterday. Knocked the socks off the therapists' expectations. As I told them, she's always full of surprises. Two full days now of consistent lucidity and responsiveness. Here's hoping for three. I'll bring her home this afternoon. Not sure about the Depakote taper down now. If she continues as she has these days, we'll probably leave things alone. The Ritalin has been phased out. We'll see how she does with home PT. (Now Blue Cross is saying it won't authorize home therapy until it sees the NRH reports, even though it had been authorized last week and the home care agency thought it could just put things on hold until she came back from the hospital; quite ironic, B.C. wouldn't pay for NRH but now won't give her home therapy without NRH input. I don't think there will be any problem once they see the reports, which recommend it, but it's annoying because I wanted it to start up on Monday and now I'm sure it'll be mid-week probably before I can get therapists out to the apt.) Stel's next MRI is tomorrow. Send your best vibes this way. I can't help but think her significant improvement may indicate something positive going on, but I'm afraid to hope, given how many times my expectations have been crushed. Love, Kay

NOTE: Even at NRH, one of the doctors lectured me on the hopelessness of Stel's diagnosis, challenging me to recite the miserable survival statistics. I was pained that the therapists bought his line and wanted to convince me I was wasting my money. I told them all that no one knows who may beat the tumor and Stel, who had many surprises in her, could be one of the survivors. In the next couple of days, she knocked them on their ears, to my great joy. I was deeply frustrated, though, that even the brain trauma experts at this first-rate hospital conveyed such pessimism.

Sun Mar 14 2000 7:54 AM

Bob, I'm amazed that in Anchorage you could find neuro-psychologists. So far, here I've found one. I expected she would know a lot about people with brain tumors since she had worked at the National Rehab Hospital, but she didn't seem to and seemed to believe that because Stel has a bad prognosis, there's not much that can be done. At any rate, she didn't recommend anyone else who might be able to work with her either. Stel has now had three or four different speech therapists and I've yet to see much progress made. Stel is pretty resistant to much of the basic stuff they do, and she really has to relate to the person well for them to be able to get her to cooperate. Anyway, I'll keep trying. I'm going to call one of the authors of the book Retraining Cognition and see whether he can refer me to someone. It's very encouraging to know about your experience, and I'm going to tell Stel about it. As we go along here, I may have more questions for you. Oh, I have one now: Did you have problems writing? Kay

Wed Mar 15 2000 6:54 AM

Barbara, I think I'm going to try to go to the meeting without Stel this time. Getting in and out of the car is just so energy-sapping for her and she'll be having physical therapy during the afternoon on Thursday. I think going out that night and sitting at a meeting for a while will be too much for her to deal with. Also, I realized I'd have to get us fed and ready in the space of an hour or two after PT, and that's more than I want to tackle. So a friend has said she'll come over and stay with Stel, and you can just pick me up if that's okay. I really wish I could take Stel, but I think maybe it would be better to try in a couple of weeks, or in April. Kay

Wed Mar 15 2000 9:04 AM

Dr. Friedman, I'm sending the MRI taken on 3/12 to you Fed Ex today. It's basically stable. Stel is doing pretty well. Kay Loveland

Fri Mar 17 2000 8:55 AM

Deborah, I'm wondering whether you'd have time in your schedule this coming week to go to the Daumier exhibition at the Phillips with Stel and me. We've always loved his work and Stel indicated she'd like very much to see the exhibition. I could probably get her there by myself, but it's difficult these days and I feel better when I have another person along. Also, it would be more fun to have company and I know Stel would really like your company. I hope we can do this. Stel is feeling down and we've got to find some fun things to do—it's been so long since we've done anything fun. It really gives her a boost whenever she sees her good friends.

Stel did great at the rehab hospital last week. The last three days she was there, she was consistently alert. She exceeded the therapists' expectations and was a joy to behold. Since she's been home, she's not as lively and part of it is because she's feeling depressed. Gotta get her out and doing things! Hope we can make some plans this week. Thanks, Kay

NOTE: The message below refers to an e-mail forwarded by someone on the BT List from another listserve—Fight for Life—which I don't think exists any more. It was a list that focused on alternative treatments for cancer in general. This particular message was from Ron Baker, whose wife, Martha, had a baseball-sized GBM in the left frontal lobe (Stel's was in the right). She had undergone months of a chemo trial at the University of Michigan. By December 1999 her doctors had declared her case hopeless and advised her husband to place her in hospice, which he did. But he began searching for other treatments and in January 2000 flew her in an air ambulance to a clinic in Tijuana operated by the American Metabolic Institute, based in San Diego. At the time he took her there, in his words, she "could not speak, think, or move a muscle in her body. She was entirely in a vegetative state." Hospice doctors had given her only a few weeks to live. The main treatment of the Mexican clinic was a vaccine made from the tumor (if possible) or from the blood or urine of the patient. In Baker's message that I read on the BT List, he recounted how his wife, by the end of their six-week stay, had "totally regained her ability to clearly think, speak, and [was get-ting] physically stronger each day." They returned home and she was undergoing physical therapy, and "getting very close to being able to bear weight on her own and walk again," at the time of his message.

Sun Mar 19 2000 10:16 AM

Dear Ron, Your e-mail about your wife is very exciting to those of us who have loved ones in similar situations. I'd like to know, first of all, how you were able to get your wife to the clinic, given the very weak state she was in. Did you fly? If so, by what airline or other carrier? Did you go by ambulance from the San Diego airport? Also, can you tell me more about your experience at the clinic. I've looked at the website and it sounds like a very nice place to be. How did the doc-tors, nurses, and other staff treat your wife? Did you stay there with her? In decid-ing to go there did you get information from them on how many brain tumor patients they've treated and what the results have been? Where was your wife's GBM located? How big was it at the time you took her there? What other treat-ments had she undergone?

Sorry for all the questions, but I'd really appreciate as much information as you can give me. My partner is not yet at the stage where the doctors are saying take her home and wait for the end, but I can envision that day coming before too many months. The last three MRIs have been stable, but unfortunately she's not functioning well physically or cognitively. She really can't do anything for herself. Your experience at AMI makes me think I ought to try to get her there before many more rounds of chemo. I very much look forward to hearing from you. I've sent a message to AMI, too. Thanks, Kay Loveland

Mon, Mar 20 2000 8:22 AM

Thanks for the information, Ron. I want to stay in touch with you and find out how Martha is doing in the next few weeks and months. My partner is about to take a first round of Temodar, but I'm looking down the road a bit and thinking AMI may be the place to try soon. All the best, Kay

Wed, Mar 22 2000 8:27 AM

Dear Carole, Stel's been mostly out of it for the last few days. Far from the lively person she was in NRH. But this seems to be a fairly common experience. Had an arduous day yesterday because we had to go out to see the oncologist and then for postponed dental appointments. First I had to deal with the car situation because it's extremely difficult now to get her into and out of the Camry. I tried to take her out for a drive on Saturday and couldn't get her satisfactorily seated, even with the maintenance man's help. So I borrowed Linda's Volvo station wagon with vinyl seats for the appointments. It's a little higher up, a little more leg room, and the vinyl helped for scooting purposes. With Linda's help we got her into the car pretty well. Had no help getting her out at the doctor's office and, of course, it was pouring rain and there is no canopy at the building. But we made it, soaked. For the dental appointments, one of the volunteers who helps me met me there to help get Stel out of the car, again in the pouring rain with no canopy. Got our teeth taken care of and then took her home, where I had assistance again from the same woman. Stel held up well throughout it all but was zonked. I put her to bed and she was asleep in five seconds.

I've got to do something about the car on a more permanent basis. Am looking into trading the Camry in for another Toyota. Problem is, the larger one is vastly more money. I've just got to get something that makes it possible for us to go places more easily. Now that I can get Stel out of the building, I've got to be able to get her into the car so we can have some enjoyment occasionally, as well as get to appointments. I can keep borrowing Linda's car, but that's not the answer for the longer term. Today I hope we can get out for some pleasure. Deborah is coming over and we're hoping to go with her, in Linda's car, down to the Phillips Gallery to see the Daumier exhibit. Stel and I both love his work and, in one of her few emphatic comments in recent days, she said she would like to see the exhibition. Fortunately, the rain has pretty much stopped. Keep your fingers crossed that we can have some fun. Kay

Wed Mar 22 2000 11:48 PM

Dear Renata, Thanks for your message. The last five months have been mostly frantic and horrible. Basically, Stel can't do anything for herself now and she has great problems communicating. She's quiet a lot of the time (very different from the Stel you knew). I'm doing everything I can to find people who can help her, but what you learn is that really not much is understood about the brain and I haven't found anyone with good answers yet. It's hard to know, too, how much of her functioning difficulties may relate to the medications she's on. The last three brain scans have shown the disease to be stable, which is good, and Stel will take her third round of chemo this week. It will be a new drug that has been getting some pretty good results for some people. So far, she hasn't had any of the anticipated side effects of the chemo, but I don't know if that will hold true for this new one. Also, I think it may be possible that these poisons are affecting her in ways we can't fathom and adding to her problems. I know of a number of people who have been in as bad or worse shape than Stel—unable to walk, talk, think—who have improved a great deal, so I have hope that she will too if the treatments work. She's done remarkable things up to now and I suspect has some more surprises in store for us. She's a sweetheart, and my heart just breaks to see her this way and having to endure what she has. It gets pretty lonely for me these days, not having Stella to talk to and share so much with. It's just a terrible struggle, but some people do beat the odds and we're fighting every inch of the way.

To answer your question: No, neither of our families are of any help with money. Fortunately, we have a few friends who are helping out financially. I'm trying to get as much assistance at home as I can through a couple of volunteer groups, friends, and probably some paid help. That will, hopefully, free up some time that I need for further research on treatments as well as my own work, and give my back a break. I've found that I'm remarkably strong, but my body was beginning to feel the strain a couple of months ago.

I wish I had better news, but it's not the worst news, either. Our mantra is "Stella is getting better," and I believe she will. Wish we could be planning to see you, but there's no way we can take any trips unless Stel is able to do more for herself. I just pray we'll have a chance to get back to Europe again together. We love it so much. Please stay in touch. Love, Kay

Fri Mar 24 2000 7:34 AM

Dr. [Alex] Spence [U of Washington]: A friend of mine attended the brain tumor regional conference in Seattle a couple of weeks ago and heard you speak. She told me what you had said about using Lasix to help keep the steroid dose lower, as well as using methylprednisolone instead of dexamethasone. I asked my partner's oncologist this week about doing the same thing. Stel has a GBM and has been on dexamethasone, at least 10 mg a day and as high as 20 mg a day on occasion, since early November. The oncologist was reluctant to use Lasix because she said you need to keep a close check on potassium levels, which is difficult with Stel since she isn't very mobile right now and also her veins are mostly shot from so many blood tests, etc. over the last few months. She did prescribe a "mild" diuretic, spironolactone, for Stel which she said wouldn't pose the potassium problems. Re the methylprednisolone, the doctor didn't feel there was much difference from the dexamethasone but said she would prescribe it if I preferred.

I'd appreciate hearing your thoughts about this. What do you do about monitoring potassium levels for patients on Lasix? Is the mild diuretic likely to be effective for the purposes you've suggested? Why do you think using methylprednisolone is better than using dexamethasone? I apologize for asking all these questions. Thanks for your response, Kay Loveland

Sat Mar 25 2000 6:58 PM

Deborah, Thanks for going with us to the Phillips Wednesday. I think Stel was very happy to get out and do something "normal" and, of course, to do it with you, as was I. As I mentioned to you, I hope you'll be able to visit fairly frequently because I know how much it does for her—and we both enjoy your company. If you can possibly work her into your schedule on a regular basis, even just for brief times, that would undoubtedly be a big boost. I don't know if weekends are ever possible for you, but they're especially hard because that's when we most want to get out—especially in the spring—and most people seem to be booked up.

Speaking of getting out, are you planning to go to the lecture on the 30th about Washington-Berlin? I don't know whether Stel would want to go, but if she does, it would be lovely to meet you there. Stel takes her new chemo Sunday through Wednesday nights and, hopefully, she won't feel big side effects from it, but there's no way to know. She could be too fatigued from it to want to go out anywhere. Again thanks, Kay

Sat Mar 25 2000 11:51 PM

Kay, I use Lasix and simultaneously administer potassium at 20 milli-equivilants twice daily. This has worked well and kept patients out of low potassium troubles. The substitution of methylpred for dexamethasone may modestly help the weakness that steroids can cause in the hip muscles. Methylpred causes all the other steroid problems that dex does—fat cheeks, increased blood sugar. The only way to get rid of the unwanted steroid effects is to get rid of the steroids, something that can only be done if the tumor volume is small enough to allow it. Thanks for your interest. Doc Spence

Sat Apr 01 2000 1:12 AM

Friends [on the BT List], I don't think it does any of us a service to dismiss a message like the one from Ron Baker as fraudulent or from a terribly misguided soul who has been taken in by the quacks in Tijuana. I was surprised to see responses that simply lumped all Tijuana, and probably most alternative, clinics into one category of quackery and fraud with no indication that anyone had ever really done any research on the particular one Baker took his wife to. I was also surprised and disheartened to see that many responders obviously hadn't read Baker's message closely. If they had, they would have seen that he and his wife had already been through ten months of a mainstream clinical trial and she was in a hospice and had been written off by the doctors when Baker decided to take her to Tijuana. The sense I have from the responders is that they don't believe what he says because they think he's fronting or shilling for the organization. Why don't people who have experiences with alternative treatments they want to share have as much right to sing the praises of these doctors and treatments as people do who extol mainstream doctors and treatments—without being labeled fronts or gullible fools? I know there are plenty of quacks and frauds out there, but I don't believe every alternative clinic or practitioner falls into that category and I don't believe that every person who goes to them should be dismissed without serious consideration of what they report about their own experience. If mainstream medicine had a great track record in coming up with effective treatments for brain tumors, maybe I could buy the argument that no one in their right mind should turn to alternative approaches. That's not the reality. As we know, mainstream treatments have pretty dismal statistics and, on top of it, the treatments can cause all kinds of additional serious problems for patients. There's plenty of suffering, for patients and caregivers, that goes on as a result of conventional treatments.

As to Ron Baker, I can only report to you that he is a real person, with a real wife named Martha, who is now in physical rehabilitation in Michigan. I spoke to him on the phone for more than an hour today. He is an ordinary person with a job who was highly skeptical of any treatments other than the mainstream until he reached the point where he had to choose either to accept the verdict of the doctors at the University of Michigan to let his wife die or to look for other alternatives. He seems to have made the right decision if one thinks it's better that his wife is now alive and on the verge of walking again rather than dead. She was in the blood-brain barrier clinical trial with carboplatin (and methotrexate, which she was on for most of the trial) at the university for ten months. Last summer she was doing extremely well, the tumor had shrunk and she was off Decadron. The doctors told the Bakers that if she started getting weaker, they shouldn't worry; it was likely a result of the treatment. She did get weaker and by the end of November she was in such bad shape that the doctors told them, to their great shock, that they couldn't do anything more for her and she should be sent to a hospice. Baker contacted Dr. Keith Black to see whether he might be able to operate on the baseball-sized tumor in the left frontal lobe (it had been declared inoperable from the beginning). Dr. Black said he couldn't do it; he didn't think she would survive the operation. Baker then began looking for other options, a sane decision in my opinion. As of now, he has his wife; he isn't bankrupt (Blue Cross paid for a large part of the treatments and tests); and he and his wife are looking forward to the future. I think it's our loss if we sneeze at this story.

I'll close with some quotes from Michael Lerner's excellent, well-researched, thoughtful book, Choices in Healing, about evaluating unconventional cancer therapies: "For almost 50 years, mainstream opponents of unconventional cancer therapies successfully portrayed unconventional therapies to the American public as practiced largely by unethical 'quack' practitioners, cynically exploiting the fears of patients for personal profit. The patients who used these therapies were portrayed as desperate and credulous people too ignorant to make informed choices. These stereotypes have proved to be highly inaccurate.

"The studies of Barrie Cassileth, Ph.D., and my own more journalistic surveys, suggest that, for the most part, unconventional therapies in the United States are offered by licensed physicians or other credentialed health care practitioners who believe in the therapies they offer, who are not charging excessive fees for treatment, and who are treating patients of above-average education. These patients are likely to be more deeply engaged than the average patient in their fight for recovery. In the large majority of cases, these patients also, significantly, choose to remain under the care of a mainstream physician.

"In my experience, patients genially leave mainstream medicine completely only because their doctors told them they had 'nothing more to offer them,' or because they had shockingly poor experience with mainstream medicine, or because they weighed the risks and benefits of what mainstream medicine offered and decided to explore other options.

"The vast majority of cancer patients do not see conventional and unconventional therapies as an either-or proposition.... It is also important to recognize that the problem of impaired physicians is as real in conventional medicine as the problem of quack practitioners is in unconventional medicine [as my partner Stel and I found out to our great shock and sadness last year]. It is my opinion, based entirely on my own personal experience, that unethical and impaired practitioners probably represent a somewhat larger proportion of unconventional than of conventional practitioners, largely because the field of unconventional therapies is unregulated and, given its socially marginalized position, probably attracts disproportionate numbers of both highly committed ethical practitioners and unethical quack practitioners."

Lerner concluded that there is little scientific evidence for most unconventional therapies "on which to evaluate questions of whether these therapies sometimes result in survival advantage, life extension, or improved quality of life," but "there is significant anecdotal or case evidence that some people have recovered from life-threatening cancers or lived for an unexpectedly long time while using many of these therapies, and that some of these therapies do enhance quality of life." I think we'd all do well to judge people's experiences with alternatives on the facts as we can ascertain them. Kay

Mon Apr 03 2000 1:53 PM

Friends [on the BT List], For the past four days, since she took her last Temodar pill, Stel has been really zonked out, sleeping most of the day and night. I'd welcome hearing of others' experience with this fatigue. How long did it last? Thanks, Kay

Mon Apr 03 2000 2:01 PM

Dear Cathy, I'd appreciate it if you could try to contact Dr. Randall Chestnut, Director of Neurotrauma and Neurosurgical Critical Care at the Oregon Health Sciences University. I saw him on a TV program on the brain yesterday and he spoke about the need for acute caregivers like surgeons to help the patient make a smooth transition to rehabilitation specialists. I'd like very much to know if he could suggest the best places he knows of for physical and cognitive rehab for people suffering from brain trauma. If you get him, tell him Stel has a glioblastoma, but she's been stable for three months. Basically, she has a lot of left-side neglect and weakness, as well as significant cognitive difficulties with memory and communication, and I've yet to find a place in this area (other than the National Rehab Hospital, which is extremely expensive and very difficult to get into) that provides good intensive rehab for people with brain injuries. I'm willing to take Stel wherever the best places are and would like his input. Thanks. Kay

Mon Apr 03 2000 10:41 PM

Kay, The Temodar fatigue could last a week more or less. I'm not sure how strong Stel is in her essential being, but it knocks me from about day 4 (first pills are Day 1) till sometime around Day 11-14. Love, Peggy

Tue Apr 04 2000 12:15 AM

To Mr. Wright [on the BT List]: You wrote, "To Mr. Baker, who is promoting this stuff, if your loved one really has a malignancy, do her a service and get her into treatment with a reputable medical center and competent specialists." You clearly didn't read his message or mine or you would know that his wife was in a clinical trial at the University of Michigan for ten months. After the doctors there gave up on her, Mr. Baker did some research and decided to take her to the clinic in Tijuana. It is not my impression from talking to him that Mr. Baker is doing anything other than telling his rather remarkable story, which he says he is still trying to absorb himself. I believe he should be able to do that without being labeled a promoter of fraudulent medicine. Sincerely, Kay Loveland

Tue Apr 04 2000 7:41 AM

Dear Ellen, Thanks so much for your messages. I am looking at the AMI thing closely. I'm talking to several patients and have a friend in California who is going to visit the facility and meet the doctor in a couple of weeks. I'd like to stay ahead of the curve of Stel's tumor if that's possible. It won't be easy to make the decision to do it, if I do, because of the kind of disdain and scorn so many people, including some friends, have for Tijuana clinics. And, of course, I never thought I'd be thinking seriously about it myself; but, then, that's what Ron Baker said, too. I want to hear from him in mid-April about his wife's next scan and follow what happens with her in the next several weeks.

Stel took her first round of Temodar this past week and she's completely zonked by it. Has been sleeping on and off for most of the day and night now for 3-4 days. The worst thing, though (I don't know that this is related to the Temodar) is that the last couple of days I've had hell getting her to take her pills. She either spits them back or holds them in her mouth and swishes the water around for 10-15 minutes before spitting them out or, sometimes, swallowing them. I ground them up in applesauce a couple of times and she took them, but last night she wouldn't eat the applesauce—it does taste icky, even though I did my best to camouflage the taste. I'm at my wit's end. I've solved a ton of problems over these months, but can't figure out what to do about this. I can't force her mouth open—it's shut too tight—and can't make her swallow, and I can't reach her mentally to reason with her about it, although a couple of times when I've almost broken down, she has swallowed. But it's so time-consuming and energy-draining, I just can't go through this day after day. Today I think I'll get some ice cream and chocolate sauce and try to make really thick, yummy shakes to put the ground-up pills in (but some pills I can't grind up). I dunno what else to do. If you have any ideas, send them along. I'm praying maybe she'll be over this phase today, but from time to time she does have problems taking pills. And I don't know what I'll do if she's still doing this kind of thing when the next round of Temodar comes up at the end of the month. I was terrified to give the pills to her this last time, and she did have trouble the first night.

Speaking of chemo, I found one of the articles posted to the List very interesting—about the mental effects of chemo. I think there's no doubt it's had and is having significant effects on Stel. This is short-term. What about the long-term, if we can get there? By the way, I finally talked to Dr. Helenowski. He said he didn't see any reason from the scans why Stel should not be doing better; said these kinds of results could happen from the radiation, but he hadn't seen it before and said one fellow who was walking fine before the procedure and couldn't walk afterwards was found to have problems with the Dilantin he'd been put on. Once that was taken care of, he walked fine again. He thinks Stel's problems are probably more related to the anti-seizure and other meds she's on and maybe to metabolic problems, like thyroid. I asked him to write a letter to the oncologist to this effect. [He never did.] I'm tired of being the message carrier between doctors. Now I want to find a different neurologist and see what adjustments can be made. Actually, I just discovered yesterday a center for Neuro-Rehab which looks promising. There, I can get the services of a neuro-psychiatrist, along with others. Trouble is they're moving their office and won't be open there until May 1. But I couldn't manage to get Stel there right now anyway. Hugs to you and Bobby. Keep on keeping on, and call whenever. Kay

Wed Apr 05 2000 5:58 AM

Dear Melinda, Re your question about Ritalin, my partner was on it for a while. The first few days she was taking it (5 mg), she was very lively and talkative. She seemed to have few word-finding problems and could converse much more as she would have before all this. But after a few days, it didn't seem to have that effect on her any more and she reverted to her mostly uncommunicative state. The doctor boosted the Ritalin to 7.5 mg a day, but that didn't appear to have any effect. After another couple of weeks, we took her off it altogether because it didn't seem to be helping and some doctors thought it could be a possible factor in seizures. The day she was off it entirely, she once again became very lively and talkative and stayed that way for about four days. She hasn't been that way since. I tried an experiment one day by giving her 5 mg of Ritalin again, since I still have a supply, but it didn't have any noticeable effect. Kay

Wed Apr 05 2000 11:38 PM

Dear Kay, Thanks for sharing your experience with Ritalin. I was wondering how Stel is doing with her speech problems. Does it ever get worse and then get better? My brother went from having some hesitation in his speech to word finding problems to stuttering and now an inability to respond with anything but yes or no (in about two weeks' time). Occasionally, he will get out someone's name but that is about it. He indicated to the doctor that he had thoughts in his head, knew the words he wanted to say but then couldn't say them. (The doctor gave three scenarios of speech difficulty and that is what he chose.) His tumor has been stable since November '99; he just switched from carboplatin to Temodar. I noted Stel is on Temodar. Do you think that the Temodar had anything to do with the speech difficulties? Thanks, Melinda

Thu Apr 06 2000 7:23 AM

Melinda, I have hope that Stel will recover a lot of her speech abilities because I've seen her "emerge" for as much as four days and be much more animated and lucid, with far fewer word-finding problems. Unfortunately, that doesn't happen very often, but it lets me know she's still there and still capable of making those connections at times. It's very possible that a good bit of the problem is related to medications, I think. I talked last week to the doctor who did the stereotactic radiation in December and he said he really didn't believe most of the problems were caused by radiation. He suspects medication and metabolic causes. I haven't gotten the doctors yet to really focus on this, but I will. I'm going to find a neuropsychiatrist and have him/her look at Stel's anti-seizure meds and see about adjustments. (I suspect Depakote.) With the Temodar, I do think she's having a little more difficulty talking in the last few days—she stutters and just can't seem to get words out or they come out very garbled. Of course, she's been so zonked, that could be the reason. We'll see as she gets a little more alert, which I believe started last night. I wish she could at least let me know whether she's got the thoughts in her head, but neither I nor the speech therapists have been able to get that kind of information out of her. She seems to have a lot of trouble making choices among options, so that doesn't work. Mostly, she's a sphinx and I just don't know what's going on in that poor battered brain, but I feel sure it's more than appears on the surface.

Not having Stel to talk to about everything is a great loss. We enjoyed that so much. On the few days and hours when she's more her old self, I'm overjoyed. It's so wonderful to have her back. I'm hoping there will be more of those days and less of the sphinx-like ones in the future. Please keep me posted on your experiences. Thanks, Kay

Thu Apr 06 2000 11:25 PM

Dear Melinda, Re your questions: (1) I don't know yet whether Temodar is working for Stel. She just had her first round last week. The doctor wants to take a scan after second round, which won't be until mid-May. Makes me nervous. (2) Stel can't get around okay. She really can't do anything for herself, can't initiate anything right now, and certainly can't walk. She's stronger than she was in January and can stand up pretty well most of the time, but walking is a real challenge. No doctor has given me any good explanation for all her problems, but I think the steroid has had a lot to do with her inability to walk—weak hip muscles and knees that buckle. She's tapering down and is now at 8 mg a day. I'm praying she'll be able to get off this time. Every time she gets this low, something happens and the doctor boosts it back up. But if she has to go back up, this time I'm asking for methylprednisolone instead of Decadron. Heard about it from a doctor in Seattle who thinks the methylpred is easier on hip muscles. (3) The stereotactic radiosurgery was done by Dr. Tomasz Helenowski at the Chicago Institute of Neurosurgery and Neuroresearch. (Stel's tumor wasn't as large as many but it was larger than most gamma knife or SR doctors will do.) He did it one-shot with the Peacock machine. Because he was using the Peacock, which is the most sophisticated machine for aiming radiation only at the places you want it to go, I wasn't worried about the one-day aspect. Now I wish we'd gone to Staten Island instead for the fractionated because Stel hasn't functioned at anywhere near the same level since the radiosurgery and I think the one massive dose may have been too much for her, even though the doctor doesn't believe radiation caused the problems. He thinks it's medications and metabolics. I've been trying to get something done about anti-seizure meds for some time and haven't accomplished it yet. I will soon and we'll see. I hope with all my heart that it does make a signifi-cant difference because I'm terrified the radiation has damaged her seriously for good. Who knows? No one can give you answers in this upside-down world we're living in. Kay

Thu Apr 06 2000 11:47 PM

Dear Carole, Stel has been really knocked out for the last week from the Temo-dar. She was a little more alert today but still pretty zonked. Given her state, she hasn't been able to do any therapy this week. Occupational therapist put her on hold and physical therapist cancelled visits this week. It looks likely that Blue Cross won't be willing to pay for any more at-home therapy right now unless there are dramatic improvements next week. It's a catch-22. She needs the ther-apy to get stronger so she can make progress, but BC won't let her have it unless she makes progress. Not sure what the next move is. I have been in touch with a Center for Neuro-Rehab in Silver Spring that looks promising. But I've got to solve the transportation problem. PT was supposed to work with us and the transfer board, but couldn't do it this week because Stel wasn't up to it. We'll do that next week and see if it is a workable solution. Stel's having a lot of trouble talking, when she tries, which isn't often. I think it may be related to the chemo, too; she's just so out of it. But who knows. It rips my heart up.

A home health aide comes five days a week in the morning and gets Stel cleaned up and helps with breakfast. At least one volunteer comes each day for three-plus hours. Stel is on the waiting list for in-home aide from Montgomery County and they said they would try to expedite it. Still waiting to hear from Montgomery County Respite Care program. [I never heard from either of these again.] Stel's friend, Cathy, from Portland is coming Saturday for three days. Until later, Kay

Sat Apr 08 2000 5:13 PM

Dear Friends [on BT List], I wondered if anyone else has had to deal with sores on the feet. Stel has developed a huge—and I mean huge—blister on the heel of her left foot. Neither doctor nor nurse seemed overly concerned about it when I mentioned it early last week. They just said to keep her heel elevated so it doesn't get more pressure put on it. Blue Cross, however, authorized the nurse to come weekly to check on it. Yesterday, the nurse put an Exuderm bandage on it and said to put another one on if it breaks and starts oozing. Now I see two red spots on each of her ankles, both of which, especially on the left, are swollen. That's how the blister started. I'm doing my best to keep her feet from touching anything, but it's not easy. If others have dealt with this problem, I'd like to know how it's been treated by other doctors and what people did to try to help the sores heal or to avoid them. Thanks, Kay

Sun Apr 09 2000 12:23 AM

Dear Deborah, Stel was pretty knocked out for more than a week as a result of the chemo. She mostly slept. The last couple of days, she's been much more alert and responsive. Her friend Cathy arrived tonight and will be here until Wednesday afternoon, and Stel's looking pretty happy to see her. Give a call when you want to come by. Thanks, Kay

Sun Apr 09 2000 11:17 AM

Kay, My wife had the same "blister" on the heel of the left foot and it broke and she's had a real sore with bleeding, etc. The nurse said at first to leave the wound uncovered and let it air out but at the end of a week they were back to dressing it with an antibiotic salve and non-stick bandages. After that week, the nurse said it looked bad and suggested a physician home visit. We called a podiatrist who removed the center and prescribed some type of boots that would prevent any further pressure while she remains in bed. We need the boots for both feet now. Hope this will not discourage you. Maybe a podiatrist is the answer. Don't wait too long. Mark Richards

Sun Apr 09 2000 6:17 PM

Mark, Thanks for your reply. We've had a nurse here who has put a dry dressing on the blister. Today I called him because it appeared Stel's ankle was red and swollen. He said he thinks this may be an infection, cellulitis, from the blister. He called the doctor's office and they prescribed an antibiotic. Stel started taking that today and I hope it will be effective. We're also awaiting the booties. I'm holding my breath that we'll nip this in the bud. Thanks for the tip about a podiatrist. I'll kegep that at the ready. Kay

Sun Apr 09 2000 6:31 PM

Charles, We're awaiting the booties that are supposed to protect Stel's feet from blisters—wish someone had mentioned them earlier. I just hope this will stop the thing before it gets worse. Could be a difficult problem to treat. Also, of course, this makes it very difficult to try to get her out to go anywhere—can't get shoes on her feet. If it's not one thing, it's three. A friend is here from the West Coast for three days. It's great to have her, but the time is too short. Thanks for your continuing concern. Kay

Mon Apr 10 2000 9:20 AM

Kay, I think you are right to be concerned about Stel's heel. Here's what happened to my mother: She's paralyzed on the left side but experienced tone problems (an up and down motion) with that leg. While in bed, this would rub her ankle on the sheets. The rubbing caused a sore, which my mom watched quietly until one morning when the whole area (and then some) became very swollen and inflamed. The area had become infected, and they put her on some antibiotics. The antibiotics caused big bouts of diarrhea. The wound failed to heal and she developed a staph infection, so she's on more antibiotics. She's also taking yogurt and acidophilus to fend off diarrhea and other antibiotic-related problems. I hope you can get Stel's blisters under control before it becomes a problem like my mom's. This all began a month ago and it's still not fully resolved. Barbara

Mon Apr 10 2000 5:58 PM

Barbara, Thanks for the info. I hope we can stop this thing before it gets so bad, but it annoys me greatly that no one mentioned getting protective booties as a preventive for this kind of thing. She started taking an antibiotic yesterday. I pray it won't lead to diarrhea, which would be a very big mess for me to deal with. Kay

Tue Apr 11 2000 8:05 AM

Kay, I did forget that my mom was later fitted for a plastic boot that helps eliminate further rubbing of the bad area. The boot looks similar to a white ski boot with velcro. My mom's diarrhea was mostly likely due to a longer course of antibiotics. Give Stel lots of yogurt, and perhaps the doctor can prescribe some powdered nystatin, both used to support the good antibodies that are diminished by the antibiotics. I'm glad to hear Stel's on antibiotics, so this thing doesn't get worse. Is Stel talking more? My mom got very quiet around the time of the diarrhea. We just assumed that when she got better she'd be back to her old self, but that's not the case. We get few words out of her a day. Barbara

Tue Apr 11 2000 10:05 PM

Barbara, Thanks for the further info. I haven't heard of a plastic boot. The ones we're supposed to get tomorrow are lamb's wool, I think. So far, so good re the diarrhea. Stel has been pretty quiet and unresponsive for several months, but she's had periods when she's much more talkative. And she often surprises me with something she'll say or something she'll laugh at. I've been searching for the right cognitive trainers. It's so frustrating not to be able to get any good answers from doctors and others regarding what may be causing the difficulties (since it doesn't appear to be tumor growth) and whether it may get better. I have hope that it will since I see those flashes of near-normalcy. I hope you find the same. Kay

Thu Apr 13 2000 7:33 AM

Carole, Stel's taking the antibiotic. The foot doesn't look worse, maybe a little better. We now have the lamb's wool booties. So far so good with the rest of her body. I do try to put her in different positions when she's in bed, but there's been no training on this score. I'll talk to the nurse. Kay

Thu Apr 13 2000 11:36 PM

Dear Ron, I'm thinking of you as the date for Martha's MRI approaches. Please let me know as soon as you can what it shows. (Stel has one scheduled for that day, too, and I'm a little apprehensive. I'm hoping it shows stability again, at least. I'll be really worried if it looks like it's beginning to grow once more.) I've spent the last couple of weeks talking to other AMI patients, to the doctor, and alternative therapy researchers, and getting other information wherever I can. As I have, I've become more and more convinced that there is something significant going on there and that Stel should be there. I've tentatively scheduled May 1st as the day to take her down. A friend of mine is going to Tijuana next Wednesday. He'll meet the doctor and see the facility and give me a report back. I'll feel better having his eyewitness report to add to yours and others. Hope everything continues to go very well and that Martha is up and about. All the best, Kay

Thu Apr 13 2000 11:47 PM

Dear Kay, Just a quick note to see how you and Stel are doing. My brother is not doing that well. We did go ahead with the Ritalin since we felt he really had nothing to lose if there was even the slightest possibility that he could get some speech back. His doctor was sure that the risk of seizures was minimal. (Two hours after the first dose he had a seizure, but I'm not sure it was related). Did you ever get speech therapy for Stel? Do you think her speech has improved at all? It is so much worse to know someone you love may be thinking of things that they want to say or ask and they can't. Fred goes for his Temodar blood work tomorrow and I hope we can get him there; he is so weak. Melinda

Fri Apr 14 2000 6:45 AM

Dear Melinda, Thanks for your note. I'm sorry to hear that your brother is so weak. Stel was like that back in January and it was very, very difficult. She's stronger now and is doing okay, given the many deficits she has. So far no improvement in speech. Every so often she surprises me with things that come out, but much of the time she's quiet or stuttering out words that I can't figure out, much to my chagrin. It is terrible to think she's trying to communicate and can't. She has had several speech therapists over the past months, but I haven't been satisfied that any of them really knew how to deal with the problems she has. I've continued to search for the right cognitive retrainer. Hang in there. I've heard of people in much worse shape than Stel or your brother who have regained a lot of their functioning. Where the brain is involved, no one really knows what may happen. Best, Kay

Sat Apr 15 2000 12:47 PM

Kay: Since talking to you Martha has continued to progress each day and just this last week she was up walking on the parallel bars with some minor assistance. We are all very optimistic about what the MRI will show Monday. I will write you next week to give you an update. Hope to meet you in May at AMI. Sincerely, Ron Baker

Sat Apr 16 2000 7:59 AM

Cathy, Just got a message from the man in Michigan whose wife is alive and well in rehab after Mexico. He said she has continued to progress each day and this week was walking on the parallel bars with a little assistance. Sounds great to me. I've made the plane reservations to San Diego for May 1st. Right now I've booked the return for June 19th, thinking if Stel does well we probably would stay in So. Cal. and visit some friends for a few days. Stel has her MRI scheduled for 12:30 PM on Monday, so at 9:30 in Portland send all your best energy Stella's way. I pray it will look no different—or better—than the previous ones. If it looks like there's new growth, I'm going to be terrified.

The last three nights have been hell getting Stel to bed. During the day she is able to stand up pretty strongly—she stood yesterday for about 5 minutes with the help of Linda and another volunteer. But each of the last three nights when I've been transferring her to bed, she's practically collapsed on me and I've struggled like crazy to keep her from going down on the floor and then to get her arranged properly in bed. So far I've managed, while cursing the gods that visit more troubles on us. Her blister looks better, but a friend sent me information on how to treat them and I'm pissed with the doctor and nurse. They've both said dry dressings and the nurse hasn't done anything about cleaning it with a saline solution or anything. The literature says a dry dressing isn't good. Needs to be moist, needs to be cleaned with saline and have one of a number of different kinds of medications applied. Shit. You try to do your best, get the knowledgeable people to tell you what to do to prevent worse things, and this is what you get. I've got to be the doctor, the nurse, the therapist, the caregiver, the everything. This morning I'm going to the pharmacy to get saline solution and whatever else I can get to put on it and I'm going to let the doctor and nurse know what I think.

I'll let you know how it goes on Monday. I should be hearing early next week about the results of the MRI scan for the woman in Michigan, who also has one on Monday. Until then, Kay

Sun Apr 16 2000 9:33 AM

Hello everyone [on BT List], I've been a little bit of a lurker on the list lately just because I haven't had the energy to be more involved. My heart goes out to all of you in the middle of this surreal thing called a brain tumor. Here is my question: Has anyone had any experience with a BT patient being unable to bend at the waist? Trying to sit Tom in his wheelchair or toilet is like trying to sit the statue of David. We can't figure out why this would be happening. More than likely it is neurological, as valium doesn't seem to have any effect in relaxing him. It went away for about a month but now seems to be returning. Any suggestions? Shelly

Sun Apr 16 2000 10:34 PM

Shelly, Yes, Stel has had this problem. It was really bad about three months ago. Then it got better. Now in the last few days she's had several times when she can't seem to bend. I don't know the reason. I couldn't link it to any medications. Must just be a result of the condition. Kay

Sun Apr 16 2000 11:32 pm

Hi Kay, I just wanted to write a quick note to say that I'd been thinking of you and Stel. This weekend I've been reading the first volume of Blanche Weisen

Cook's biography of Eleanor Roosevelt. I remember how Stel told me how well written the work was, and how much of a refreshingly feminist perspective Cook takes. We also talked about how CUNY might be a good place for me with people like Cook here. Although I haven't been able to take a class with her, there have been so many wonderful professors here who seem to have similar perspectives, including my advisor. I just wanted to let Stel know that, thanks to her encouragement and wise advice, I feel like I've found my niche. Love, Beth

Mon Apr 17 2000 6:30 PM

Dear Beth, Thanks for sending your message. I will read it to Stel. You underscored two of Stel's most wonderful attributes—her encouragement and wise advice to her friends about a wide range of things. She has a generosity of spirit that is extremely rare and has always been a great source of inspiration and support to those of us lucky enough to be her friend. That was a great strength of hers, as well, when she was a teacher. The silence of her voice and concern is a great loss for all of us, but I hope the day will come when the Stella who has given us so much will re-emerge and we can all tell her how much we missed her. Love, Kay

Tue Apr 18 2000 6:52 AM

Dorothy, When you say your husband had "medically intractable partial simple seizures," what are you referring to? Stel has a lot of shaking of her left leg and arm, and sometimes her right, which I can usually stop by pressing hard on the joints. Sometimes the shaking persists longer than other times. She usually shakes when she tries to stand up or when her foot gets in certain angles when she's sitting. The doctor said these are tremors, not seizures because I can stop them, and that was my view of them, too. The physical therapist said they result from Stel's muscle weakness. A couple of months ago Stel had an EEG to look for continuing seizures and the neurologist found none. But I'm wondering whether there's more here I should look into. I want someone who understands the medications to coordinate them. Maybe an epileptologist is the answer? Kay

Tue Apr 18 2000 7:16 AM

Dear Gail, Good to hear from you. I can't imagine how you tracked me down, but I'm glad you did. As I told you on the phone, life here is pretty tough right now. There are many terrible things about dealing with a brain tumor. One of them is that life becomes completely unpredictable. That is certainly the way it's been for most of the last year. For the past 3-4 months Stel has really been unable to do anything for herself, so the caregiving duties have become completely around the clock, and there aren't any family members on either side who can, or will, be of much help. As much as I hate seeing Stel in this circumstance, I treasure every moment with her and everything I can do for her. For thirty-plus years, our greatest pleasure has been being together and that hasn't changed. I believe it is possible that Stel will regain a lot of her functioning, but it's a long, hard, terrifying road.

Thanks again for tracking me down. I look forward to the day when we can see each other under happier circumstances than the present. All the best, Kay

Tue Apr 18 2000 7:49 PM

Dear Ron, Stel's MRI looks basically stable. The radiologist thought it might have increased in size slightly. There is more swelling, he said, than a couple of months ago. I'm relieved the scan didn't show any significant increase—and I think, just looking at it myself, that the radiologist may not be right about any increase. Of course, I would be happiest to see shrinkage. I hope we'll see that, as you did, after a few weeks in Mexico. I'm eagerly awaiting word of the results of Martha's scan. Kay

Tue Apr 18 2000 11:50 PM

Kay: MARTHA'S SCAN SHOWS ANOTHER 25-30% TUMOR SHRINKAGE FROM HER SCAN DONE IN MEXICO. THIS MEANS IT IS 85-90% GONE FROM HER DECEMBER SCAN THAT WAS TAKEN BEFORE SHE WAS SENT TO HOSPICE. THIS HAS BEEN AN INCREDIBLE DAY!! Ron Baker

Wed Apr 19 2000 6:25 AM

Ron, Fantastic news!! I pray Stel will follow in Martha's footsteps soon. I will call you in the next few days. Thanks for the wonderful news. Kay

Wed Apr 19 2000 6:42 AM

Cathy, Just got the message below from the man whose wife was at death's door in December. Fantastic, isn't it? I'm anxious to get Stel down there ASAP. Wish I could have made the reservation for next week, but there's so much I've got to take care of beforehand. Re Stel's MRI, the radiologist's report said he thought there was slight growth. Could be, but comparing the scan to the one taken at the end of December (which the radiologist didn't have), they look very much the same to me. He did say there was more swelling, which I thought, too. Stel has been very sleepy and lethargic the last couple of days and I think that may be the reason for it. She's tapered down to a low steroid dose (4 mg) and it may be too low so I did what the doctor would do and upped the dose a bit, much as I hated to. Hopefully, it will help her. I also saw on the BT list a number of people talking about how problems related to speech and cognition and movement had been caused by swelling. Could be the case with Stel, as well. Her foot looks pretty good. I hope we can get it sort of back to normal before we leave. Thanks for your message and good thoughts, and Viva Mexico!! Kay

Wed Apr 19 2000 7:36 AM

Dear Ellen, Glad to get your message the other day. I've been in a whirlwind here. What I'll write to you in this message I DON'T WANT TO GO TO THE BT LIST because I know the reaction I would get from many people on it. I want to wait until there are results to report, so keep this info to yourself for now. Over past weeks I've continued to research the Mexico connection and after a lot of talking to people and other investigation have decided to take Stel there. We're going on May 1st, accompanied by her cousin. Half a dozen of our friends are highly supportive. I haven't told the rest yet, most of whom I'm sure will think I've lost my mind, along with the doctors who have yet to be told. Maybe so, but I don't think so. I just got a message from Ron Baker about his wife's MRI on Monday. The scan showed it's 85-90% gone from the scan in December. His wife is continuing to make progress toward walking. If things go for Stel as they went for Martha Baker, we'll probably be down there about six weeks. I'm convinced, Ellen, that the doctor there has something in his vaccine, which he's been using for about fourteen years. A recent quote I saw from Keith Black at Cedars Sinai about "teaching white cells to attack the tumor" could have come directly out of Dr. Rubio's mouth. So we're not talking esoteric treatments here. In addition, I like their holistic approach. They don't just deal with the tumor; they deal with the whole person. A friend is going to the clinic today for a consultation with Dr. Rubio.

Having talked to two other GBM patients who had been given months to live at Mayo and in New Brunswick before they went to the clinic eight and fourteen years ago, as well as to Baker, I believe Stel has a good chance of being a survivor. Would I like to have the results of clinical trials that assure me that is the case? Of course. But since those aren't available, one has to gather all the info one can in other ways and make the best judgment one can. That's what I've done. Given that all the treatments available for GBM now are crapshoots, I really don't think this is more of one than continuing on Temodar or some other godawful chemo. I know, all we have are anecdotes, but at the moment I'm throwing in our lot with the anecdotes instead of waiting on the clinical trials, and I have no reason now to think that Stel won't benefit from that decision. As you know, it's a horrible, terrible responsibility to bear, but one we all try to exercise in the best way we can. Just as Ron Baker said, I never thought I'd be going to a clinic in Tijuana, but as we all know, struggling to beat this terrible disease takes you down many paths you never dreamed you'd try. If, god forbid, it doesn't work for Stel, I think there's time to bring her back to the mainstream. She had a scan on Monday that is basically stable again.

Stel can't communicate very well right now, but she's managed to let me know that she's glad I've taken this course and believes it is the right one. Every day when I give her new, hopeful information, her eyes light up, though she's an even greater skeptic than I and I think can't quite give herself over to the idea that she could actually get well

I hope you and Bobby are doing as well as possible and having some happy times, despite the big hole in your lives right now. Send your best vibes toward Mexico as we keep on keeping on! Love, Kay

Wed Apr 19 2000 11:39 PM

Ellen, Just wanted to add that when I told Stel this morning about the message from Baker, she began laughing and crying at the same time—the greatest display of emotion I've seen from her in months—and saying, "It's wonderful, it's wonderful." I told her our cry from now on is "Viva Mexico" and "Viva Stella." Our friend saw Dr. Rubio today and found him to be a very unpretentious, open, accessible, positive doctor who spent more than an hour answering questions. Chris said the place is very modest, as I knew, very clean and pleasant. I also thought of the fact that when Stel and I talked to Dr. Helenowski before the radiosurgery procedure, we never got any hard numbers or results of clinical trials from him. The most he could tell us is that he's done thousands of these procedures and he thought the risk of serious harm to Stel from the radiosurgery was minimal, with the up side being that the procedure could buy her 3-6 months of time. So not every decision we make in the mainstream world is based on hard scientific facts proven in clinical trials, either. All the best, Kay

Thu Apr 20 2000 7:42 AM

Dear Ellen, Re your comment that Temodar "really isn't that bad": Stel took her first round of Temo last month—and would have been scheduled to take another round starting April 23rd. She did okay on it except she was completely zonked out for more than a week. It's not the immediate side effects that are godawful, but the very idea that basically you're putting poison into your system—I was terrified by the warning labels about NOT GETTING THE CONTENTS OF THE CAPSULES ON YOUR SKIN since Stel has some trouble sometimes these days getting pills down and starts chewing on things she shouldn't. She did chew on the first capsule but I managed to wrest it from her mouth before she chomped so hard that she broke it. Anyway, the very idea of giving her any of these terribly toxic drugs, which can depress the immune system and cause longer term problems (assuming you're one of the lucky survivors) is godawful to her and to me. If it's not necessary because there's a less toxic, more effective way, it's even more godawful.

I agree with you that it's sobering to think that we never know how much time we have with these horrible tumors and if the Mexico treatment fails, we may have time for something else or we may not. That's the one very down side I've isolated in this decision, I don't think anything about the Mexican treatment itself is likely to be harmful to Stel. The question is time, and in the race against the beast, we never know what it's going to do and how much time we're going to have. It is a gamble. I just keep telling myself that Ron Baker's wife was in far worse shape when she arrived there and despite that, within a few short weeks, she was much better. If it worked for her, with an inoperable baseball-sized tumor in the same general location as Stel's, it seems to me likely that it will work for Stel. The GBM patient who went down there fourteen years ago with a death sentence of no more than two months was also in worse shape and had the same experience of getting better soon, as did the third GBM survivor I talked to. I'll take those odds. Besides, we have no guarantees that if she continues on Temo or other chemo drugs that they're going to be effective for her (certainly the tumor hasn't yet shrunk in the three months she's been taking CCNU and Temo) and we might well find ourselves in a frantic race against time even if we adhered to the straight and narrow path. Until later, Kay

Fri Apr 21 2000 4:06 PM

To Brain Tumor List: My wife had surgery on Monday to try to remove as much tumor as possible. She is now mostly paralyzed on her left side. There is just a tad bit of movement in her arm, and no movement in her leg. She also can't talk. Is this a normal response to a craniotomy? How concerned should I be? David

Fri Apr 21 2000 5:26 PM

David: My partner Stel couldn't move her left side at all. After two weeks in the hospital, she went to sub-acute rehab where she had physical and occupational therapy every day and she walked out of rehab in twelve days with a quad cane. Soon thereafter she was walking without any cane and with minimal assistance from me. She was also using her left arm/hand pretty well. Your wife may do the same thing. Kay

Fri Apr 21 2000 6:06 PM

Dear Friends, Today is the one-year anniversary of the beginning of this night-mare Stel and I have been living. After arguing with myself for a couple of days, I've finally decided that the best way to communicate the significant news I have to tell you is by e-mail. I'd like to call each of you personally to tell you of the decision I've made and everything I went through over the past five weeks to come to it, but I have neither the time nor the energy to do that. So e-mail will have to serve as a proxy for those conversations for now. I've also decided that I can conserve my limited time and energy even more by sending you a copy of the message I faxed to Stel's oncologist yesterday. It doesn't tell you everything, but the essence is there. It is copied below.

I'll just say further that I'm very excited and hopeful about the treatment I've chosen, as is Stel and her cousin Bill, and our friend Chris, who had an hour-long consultation with the doctor Wednesday, as well as several other friends. Of course, there's trepidation and self-questioning too, as there is with every decision one makes that affects life and death. When you deal with such matters, especially in the brain tumor world, you find yourself considering many options that only a short time before would not have been within the realm of possibility—multiple craniotomies, huge radiation doses, poison in one's veins, and then you begin to look at other alternatives you never would have thought of before. The one I've chosen I think combines the best of the holistic approach with what appears to me to be good medicine and science. From everything I can gather, the doctor is a very special practitioner who for about fifteen years has been using a vaccine that works for many people with a variety of cancers, including brain tumors. Given that it's all a crapshoot at this point to find an effective treatment for a GBM, I've come to believe as I spoke to people and searched out information wherever I could that this treatment offers Stel as good a shot as she's likely to get at beating the odds and having a decent life in the process.

You've all been wonderful to Stel and me over this last year. I hope you'll hang in there with us, even if you think I've lost my mind. According to the doctor and patients I've spoken with, we'll know in a matter of 2-3 weeks max whether she is responding positively; and if she does, she should be in considerably better shape when we return home, probably in about six weeks. There will still be much to be done with physical and cognitive therapy in all likelihood, but the future will look much brighter.

If you have the time, I hope you'll drop by or call before we leave on May 1st. Here's the message I sent to the oncologist:

"Dear Doctor: I'm sorry to have to communicate with you in this way, but it seems best at the moment since telephone conversations are always so rushed and there's no time at this point to schedule a face-to-face meeting. I want to let you know that after more than a month of investigation and research I have made the decision, which Stel has indicated she agrees with wholeheartedly, to take her to a clinic in Mexico for treatment. From everything I have been able to ascertain, the doctor there has had remarkable success with brain tumors and other forms of cancer using an autologous vaccine he developed about fifteen years ago. (I understand that doctors at the University of Michigan were stunned this week to view the MRI of a patient they had given up for dead in December. The inoperable baseball-sized GBM seen on the December scan had been reduced 85-90% on the April scan.) The vaccine is used as an integral part of a holistic approach. It appears to me that the vaccine works much as those that are now being developed and tested with some encouraging results in the United States. We will be flying to San Diego, accompanied by Stel's cousin, on May 1st and will probably be at the clinic about six weeks. The doctor will know more specifically after she's been in treatment about ten days. At that stage, he says he will have a good idea of how she is responding to the treatment. I'm not sure when we will return here but I expect it will be about the middle of June if everything goes as well as we hope.

As you can imagine, this has not been an easy decision. But, then, no decision involving treatment for brain tumors is. As with others I've talked to who have gone to the clinic, I approached the idea of a clinic in Tijuana with great skepticism and am amazed to have made the decision I have. I believe, nevertheless, that it is the right one for Stel at this point and I've increasingly come to believe in the last few weeks that this treatment offers her a very good chance of getting well. Fortunately, a number of our friends agree with this decision, but I'm sure there are others who will think I've lost my mind. You may think so, too. I hope, however, that you will remain available to Stel for the follow-up portion of the treatment, if that is necessary, and for returning to mainstream approaches if she does not respond as positively to the vaccine as others have. We'll be in touch.'

Until later, friends, VIVA MEXICO! VIVA STELLA! Kay

Fri Apr 21 2000 11:28 PM

Dear Mary, I wanted to let you know what I've decided about further treatment for Stel. She took two rounds of CCNU and one round of Temodar and tolerated them okay. She had an MRI done Monday and basically it shows that the tumor is stable, as it has been for the last four months. But she's really not functioning in any meaningful way, although she's eating well and doesn't look sick.

More than a month ago I started researching the treatment given at a clinic in Tijuana and the more I learned, the more I believed there's a very special doctor working there whose vaccine and other holistic regimen is working for many cancer patients, including several with GBMs. I've decided to take Stel down there on May 1st. I haven't said anything about this on the BT List because I know the vocal people on there would have only negative things to say about it. I figure I'll wait until there are results. According to the doctor, within ten days' time he should have a good feel for whether she's responding positively and certainly by three weeks, we should know for sure. I'll copy below the message I faxed to her oncologist yesterday, which will give you the essence of the reason I've decided to go ahead with this.

I don't know whether you have any interest in pursuing treatment outside the mainstream for your sister, but I wanted you to know about this if you do. If you want me to, I'll do my best to let you know how it's going as soon as I can. Kay

Sun Apr 23 2000 7:10 AM

Dear Emily, As I said when we met a month ago, the only thing predictable about my life at this point is that it's unpredictable. This week, after several weeks of research and investigation, I've made the decision to take Stel out of town for treatment for several weeks. There is a promising vaccine that I believe may well enable her to get well, as it has for others I've spoken to. We'll be leaving on May 1st. As a consequence, I'm going to have to readjust my work schedule. I'd say I'd try to work on the book while I'm gone, but I know that is folly. What I propose is that I continue on the schedule through the end of April. Then in May I will take sick leave I have available under the Family Friendly Leave Act. I believe that will carry me to June. I don't know when I'll be back in June, so I think the best thing to do is to take that month as leave without pay. It may be that I will be able to work during the latter part of June, but that depends on when we get back and how well Stel is doing at that time. Given the uncertainties, for now I'd like to plan on taking June as unpaid leave. I hope that I can go back to the schedule we agreed on in July and make real progress on the book. Please let me know if there's anything I need to sign. Thanks so much for your support. Kay

Sun Apr 23 2000 7:59 PM

Kay, Your thoughts are right on. I look forward to news. Ellen

Sun Apr 23 2000 9:13 PM

Dear Ellen, Thanks for your note. We're counting the days until we get to Mexico. All our friends are very positive about this decision. I faxed the oncologist and neurosurgeon with the news. Didn't hear anything back. Sent an e-mail to Friedman today. Responses, or lack thereof, will be interesting. The rallying cry from now on is VIVA MEXICO! VIVA STELLA! I'll be in touch in some way. All the best, Kay

Sun Apr 23 2000 10:50 PM

Dear Kay, You are not crazy. You are thoughtful, researching, resourceful and loving without boundaries. This will work. It isn't lost on me that I received your e-mail on Easter. Your journey to Mexico for Stel's treatment may be a resurrection from the grip of this tumor. I hope so. To new life! Karen

Mon Apr 24 2000 8:09 AM

Kay, Thank you for sharing this with me. You are right to follow your feelings on this one, especially since you have been so methodical in deciding Stel's treatments. After all, we all already know chemo is not a cure, and if you strive to find something to work more than marginally, you do need to look outside of already-accepted treatments. My sister just had her two-year mark last week. We are blessed she has made it this far, but unfortunately her condition is steadily worsening. Her last MRI two weeks ago was stable, but she is increasingly childish and lethargic, and has lost a great deal of mobility. She's beginning her second round of VP-16 this week, mostly because she tolerated this very well and we do feel it is keeping things at bay for awhile. Kay, all my best wishes go out to you both. Please keep me informed how things are going. Mary

Tue Apr 25 2000 7:27 AM

Mary, I'm making contingency plans in case Stel doesn't respond positively, but deep down I believe she's got a real chance to beat the odds with this treatment. It's a gamble, but that's true of all these GBM treatments at this point. Getting her on the plane and across country isn't going to be easy, but her cousin is going to fly down with us. If ever there were a reason to put us all through this, I think this is it. At least I don't have to fly her there in an air-ambulance as the most recent BT patient did back in December.

I sent an e-mail to Dr. Friedman about my decision. He wished us well although he doesn't agree with the decision and said to keep him posted. Haven't heard anything from the local doctors. Thanks for your phone number. I'll be in touch. Kay

Tue Apr 25 2000 11:06 PM

Dear Karen and Judy, Thank you both for your messages. It's wonderful to know there's a candle at Notre Dame for Stel. That's in addition to whatever one does at the Wailing Wall, and the prayers that were offered last year by a gay group in London who found out about us through a friend visiting there, and the prayer circle one of the women at my office has enlisted, and all the other candles lit, prayers said, and just plain old good thoughts all over the place that have been directed Stel's way. I wouldn't even doubt that they might have played a part in causing the right message to come across my computer screen at the right time so I could "discover" the treatment in Tijuana. Re vaccines, there are trials going on in the states, and the description of some of them is very similar to what the doctor in Mexico is doing. When I told Stel that today, she began laughing and crying at the same time. She's so happy and relieved—as am I—to think there really is a treatment available that offers real hope of a future. Please stop by Friday evening if you can. I'll be in the throes of packing, but we'd love to see you. Kay

Sun Apr 30 2000 12:09 AM

Dear Friends, In case you want to get in touch with us during the next six weeks or so, I'm putting the phone numbers and mailing address below. We fly out of here at 1:15 on Monday. We go with a lot of hope and positive energy from all the prayers and good wishes you and others are sending our way. VIVA MEXICO! VIVA STELLA! Kay

NOTE: I wasn't able to connect my computer to the Internet at the clinic, so there are no e-mails for the seven weeks we were there. But I kept a daily journal, and I've excerpted it below.

Mexico Journal

Mon, May 1, 2000

Arrived at hospital at 5:30 PM. Stel held up fantastically well throughout the trip. She was wide awake the whole way, ate well on the plane. When we got to San Diego, the clinic van was waiting for us—but it had no wheelchair lift, so we had to get help from a young sky cap to lift her out of the wheelchair and up into the van. Once in the van, Stel sat upright and stayed awake the whole way to the clinic. When they took her out of the van and placed her in the bed in her room, she looked around with wide eyes. I'm very encouraged by her stamina through this very long, arduous day! The hospital is a tiny place in the midst of a busy business area. Stel's room is medium-sized, pleasant. There is space for a double bed for me as well as Stel's hospital bed, a large recliner, small TV/VCR, and built-in drawers and closets. The sliding glass door opens onto the patio and swimming pool. We're here!

Tue, May 2, 2000

Woke up at 7 AM. Got Stel's breakfast from the dining room—oatmeal, good toast, papaya, orange juice, parsley tea. She ate well. The nurse cleaned Stel up.

Then a doctor inserted a port in her upper right chest; he had trouble finding the vein. When he asked her name, Stel told him "Stelyani Sandris." Dr. Rubio came in later in the morning. He's young-looking, has a sweet expression. He sat down on the bed to explain the components of the treatment. He says swelling is causing a lot of Stel's problems. In ten days he thought she would be talking better and have better bladder control. He said he does low-dose radiation to "shrink and incapsulate" the tumor. This disturbed me because Stel has already had her maximum dose of radiation, plus radiosurgery. I doubt his radiation will do what he says, and I told him I was reluctant to approve that. In three weeks, she will get the main vaccine shot cultured from the tumor sample I had sent down. Stel enjoyed her lunch—quinoa, salad, fish and veggie soup, baked fish with green peppers, baked squash, hand-made tortillas, parsley tea. She had beet and carrot juice, too. In the afternoon, the nurses inserted a catheter, after the doctor persuaded me it would be best. After a good dinner, Stel went to sleep and I did, too. At 11:30 PM, I awoke because I heard Stel making noises, snorting. I leaped up and saw her contorted face, eyes rolling. She was having a convulsion. Fear grabbing my heart, I ran out to the nurse's desk and screamed, "seizure, she's having a seizure." The nurse and doctor on duty came in the room. They gave her a shot of mannitol, I think, that helped calm her down. I couldn't sleep after that, thinking I've done the wrong thing to bring her here. This is the worse seizure she's ever had. IS THIS A BIG MISTAKE??

Wed, May 3, 2000

Stel seemed okay when she woke up. I asked if she was hungry and she said "yes" emphatically. I breathed a sigh of relief. Another good breakfast that she ate with gusto. Dr. Tapia, a surgeon-oncologist came in to evaluate Stel. He will be consulting with Dr. Rubio. In the afternoon, after she was cleaned up, hospital attendants took Stel outside to the patio by the swimming pool. They insisted in carrying her out there on a sort of lounge chair, even though I told them I could get her up and into the wheelchair to take her outside. It was a beautiful day with a nice breeze. Stel was outside an hour and a half, mostly sleeping. I was excited to meet Ron and Martha Baker by the pool. She's here for a follow-up week—a vaccine booster. She still shows the effects of the steroids, but she's sitting up, talking, smiling. Her parents are here, too. It's a great inspiration to see her!

Thu, May 4, 2000

Stel had a coffee enema this morning, then the nurses cleaned her up. I gave her the oxygen therapy (she breathes from a nebulizer that I hold close to her). Dr.

Rubio won my reluctant consent to do a few radiation sessions (he says each session is only 100 rads and no patient gets more than ten sessions, some less). We had a jostling ride in an ambulance through traffic and pollution in downtown Tijuana to the hospital where the radiation equipment is. It's a very simple-looking setup, which made me nervous. While we were waiting for almost an hour, Stel threw up, mostly the beet juice she had earlier. Because of that, we left without her getting radiation. When we got back, Stel ate a good lunch. Bill (her cousin) was here and so I took a walk in the neighborhood. It's amazing how the hospital has created a small oasis only a couple of blocks from bumper-to-bumper traffic, a cacophony of noise, neon signs and stores of all kinds. Sitting in the patio of the hospital, you look up at a palm trees waving against a very blue sky and all seems calm, clean, and peaceful. When I got back, Bill had left. Stel slept a lot of the day. The Bakers came in late in the evening from a day they spent at Rosarita Beach. Martha looked relaxed and happy. I can't wait to see Stel enjoying life like that again!

Fri, May 5, 2000

Stel said "good morning" to the nurse this morning. She also laughed while watching people on TV who were screaming while riding a roller coaster! She tried talking a little more this morning and was quite alert—watching animals on TV. It's exciting! I exercised her arms and legs. The right leg was much more flexible than other days, and the right arm and hand were a little more flexible. We went for radiation today. It seemed so casual. I was nervous that Stel was placed on a narrow perch without rails or straps. She was just told to stay still. We could see her on a monitor. She moved her legs during the session. When we got back, Ron and Martha came in the room to say goodbye. Ron told Stel to believe that Dr. Rubio would turn her around as he had Martha. He hugged Stel. I hugged Martha. Stel began laughing and crying at the same time. Dr. Rubio came after that. He checked her right arm and reflexes of right foot. He said she's doing well. By Monday he thinks she should be moving more. Today she was moving her head better than he thought she would be. She should be more flexible. Her limbs were definitely more flexible today. I bent her knee normally and could rotate her feet without their becoming rigid. In the evening, Stel was talking a little more. When the nurse put a cabbage poultice on Stel's head (Dr. Rubio said this will draw radiation out), I called her a "cabbage head" and she laughed. She watched "Providence" on TV.

Sat, May 6, 2000

I tried to get Stel to talk and respond early this morning, but there was nothing. When the nurse came in, Stel laughed and repeated her "Good morning, Stella." Then we said the nurse's name (Myra), and Stel said, "Good morning, Myra." During morning exercise, Stel's left leg was more rigid than yesterday but it loosened up easily. Her left hand gripped strongly and left foot rotated easily. Same on right side. Later, another nurse asked Stel how she is. Stel responded, "fine." The nurse asked again and Stel said "fine" again. The nurse said she was putting in an IV and Stel said, "I be fine" twice. When I told Stel what she said, she laughed. For the first time, I got Stel up in the wheelchair and took her to the dining room for dinner. She sat up for two hours, but she was quite uncommunicative and lethargic. I exercised her in the wheelchair and both legs seemed more supple. Her legs weren't shaking when she was in the wheelchair. For most of today, Stel was sleepy and lethargic and mostly uncommunicative. She seemed really out of it tonight, so much so that she couldn't eat her apple, which she does most evenings. This worries me. I felt low most of the day except when Stel laughed and when I did her exercises.

Sun, May 7, 2000

Stel was unresponsive this morning—only a "Hi, Kate" out of her. Her limbs were a little stiffer but became flexible fairly easily, except for her right arm, which was still pretty rigid and her hand in a fist. I got Stel into the wheelchair for lunch in the dining room. She was very unresponsive, with a far-away look in her eyes, lethargic. When I said "the chicken is good," she said "yes," and when I said we would go outside after lunch, she responded "yes" again. We were outside for half an hour. Stel was sleeping in the wheelchair. When I put her into bed, she was very tired and almost unable to hold her head up. In the chair, her legs and arms shook, unlike last night. I'm very upset and worried. I don't see any real change—maybe she's even a little worse—so unresponsive.

Mon, May 8, 2000

In the early morning, Stel was the same as yesterday. She said "yes" a couple of times and at first looked bright-eyed, but she quickly became sleepy and was looking off in space. Her exercises were about the same as yesterday. Dr. Contreras came in at 9:15 and asked how she is. I told him she was unresponsive over the weekend. Friday was the best day. He said there would be ups and downs. In mid-day we took her for a second radiation session; she moved her head. Dr.

Tapia came in to see her later and talked to Dr. Contreras about her lethargy. I talked today to Bill Blakley, the patient who was diagnosed with a GBM fourteen years ago and came down here with two months to live, according to his doctors at home. He says the brain tumor has been gone for years and he's here now because of some spots on his lungs. He told me not to worry, that it was up and down with him for several weeks until he got the vaccine. That made me feel a little less anxious. Dr. Rubio checked Stel late in the day. He said she's doing okay. The radiation is increasing swelling, which makes her sleepy. After 2-3 more sessions, this should get better, he said. He thinks she's much less spastic. He's giving her extra mannitol for the swelling. This evening Cathy called and after I talked to her, I leaned over Stel to tell her. She looked at me and said "Kate" and something I couldn't make out, and laughed and laughed. She tried to speak a couple of more times before she went to sleep.

Tue, May 9, 2000

When Stel woke up she seemed a little brighter and seemed to smile slightly when I spoke to her. She repeated "Hi, Stella." Later she said "sweet," "now, sweet"—I think she was referring to the juice she drank. She tried to say a few words, but after breakfast she was unresponsive again. Bill Blakley came in and talked to Stel about his experience. She stared straight ahead, impassive, and never responded in the five minutes or so he talked to her. She was sleepy after that. Stel had her third radiation session today. When she looks at me, her eyes often seem beseeching, stricken, as if she's trying to speak to me. She looked at me that way, and tried to say something, when the nurses changed her catheter. It upset me a lot. All her limbs, hands and feet seemed much more normal when I exercised her this afternoon. Dr. Contreras came in and asked Stel how she is. She said, "Oh, I don't know." Stel wouldn't watch the TV. Didn't see Dr. Rubio today. I'm very down again; there's no sense Stel is responding. She did seem to be paying attention to me when she saw I was worried, but no words. I'm so worried.

Wed, May 10, 2000

Stel not talking, very sleepy all morning. I couldn't get her to say anything. Exercise—her left side was very flexible, normal; hand not grabbing; foot without clonus. The right leg loosened up quickly; no clonus in foot. Right arm and hand were more rigid and harder to loosen up. After breakfast, she was so lethargic. I couldn't get her to swallow pills and had to put them in juice. Finally, Stel spoke. I said "Stella." She said "yes." Later she said, "I wonder if…." She was fairly awake when Bill Blakley came in but just looked at him and said nothing. Dr.

Rubio checked her reflexes and said they were good and her limbs were good. He said the pressure in her brain is less because her legs and arms moved better. He asked if she responds when I speak loudly to her. I said a lot of times no. He said let's give it more time. He wants me to exercise her every two hours and try to keep her awake by pressing on her spleen and kidney or touching the bottom of her foot lightly to induce a reflex.

Later I got Stel up in the wheelchair and outside. She slept while sitting in the chair. There was no leg or foot shaking for 2 1/2 hours while she was in the chair. When I took her back inside, I kneeled down next to her and looked into her eyes. I told her how lonely I felt not being able to talk to her and asked her to say something. In a few moments, she tensed her right side, concentrated mightily, and said with effort, "My little lovebug," looking straight at me. My heart leapt and I told her how happy that made me, how much her effort meant, and tears streamed down my face. We spent another several moments looking intently into each other's eyes. I held her right hand, which was very tensed. When I transferred her to bed, she stood for a couple of minutes and straightened her knees several times. She was mostly awake until about 9 PM

Thu, May 11, 2000

This morning, the night nurse asked Stel if she was tired and she said "no." I asked her if she was hungry, and she said, "yes." As I was exercising her, she said "Wait for…" Her left arm and leg were more rigid and there was some clonus in the left foot. Her right side was pretty rigid. As I was exercising her, I told her her face had a frown and repeated, "face, face, face." She responded, "I space, space, space." I said, "I love this face." Stel said, "I love, I love." As I rubbed lotion on her nose, I said "you don't want a dried out nose." She said "no." But when the nurse came to clean her up, Stel wouldn't say hello. Later, she was looking off in space, and I thumped on her tummy and asked her where she was. She said, "Seven minutes." When I exercised her in the afternoon, I started coughing and Stel looked at me and stuttered, "What I have done?" I told her she could help me by doing her exercises and she did help with her right leg. Drs. Contreras and Tapia came in and checked her reflexes. Dr. C said she's responding whereas some people are just inert. Dr. T said it's up and down with this kind of tumor and she will probably go back and forth but get better as treatment moves along.

Later, Stel had her hand against her head. I asked, "What are you doing?" She responded, "What am I doing?" She had much more eye contact with me today and was more "with it," although still sleepy. Could it just be the effect of the small increase of Decadron? As I changed her position in bed, saying I didn't like her position, Stel said "position." She got rigid on her right side and when I asked her what's going on, she said, "He [unintelligible]…" As I was exercising her right arm, she seemed to complain, saying something like "elbow." When Dr. Rubio came in, he said she is responding well. He said her name and she turned her head and looked at him. I told him about the rigidity on her right side and how she seems to see or hear something at those times and asked whether Decadron could be causing hallucinations. He said her eyes and reflexes wouldn't be as good as they are if that's the case. It's probably the tumor structure, he said. When he left, he said, "You'll be surprised when she starts talking to you." As I got her into the wheelchair, Stel said, "Is Mrs. Dole going to…" As Stel sat in the wheelchair, we listened to music. I danced and swung her hands in rhythm. I took her to the dining room for dinner. Throughout, Stel was having right-sided rigidity spells. Her limbs were stiffer tonight when I exercised her and most of the day she had right-side rigidity. But she took all her pills today and I was able to clean her teeth with no problems.

Fri, May 12, 2000

Stel was awake early. Her eyes were bright; she was very alert and responsive with her eyes. She took all her pills well. I said "Hi" to her and asked her to say "Hi, Kate." She said "Hi." After breakfast, she got sleepy. I talked to her about how she tried so hard at the National Rehab Hospital and asked why she's not doing the same here, and why she doesn't seem to make the effort to talk to Dr. Rubio that she did with her doctors back in Maryland. (Stel's lack of any effort to respond to the nurses and the doctor here is strange. It's so unlike her.) She looked at me intently, got very rigid on her right side, looked worried, as if she wanted to speak. She abruptly started coughing, and I had to shake her. Then Stel got very sleepy. When I woke her by thumping on her tummy, she said "Ah, it's, it's…" We took her for her fourth radiation session. I'm hoping this will be the last, since that is all Martha Baker had. When we came back, I asked Stel if she was hungry. She answered, "No." She wasn't tensing up as much today as yesterday, but it may be because she's sleepy.

Dr. R said that now that she's had four rads, he can increase the aminos he's giving her and the Poly-MVA; and he can begin growth hormones to reconnect things in her brain. That troubled me and I asked whether they could cause the tumor to grow. He said it's like setting a back fire after the radiation. I asked whether he had given them to Martha Baker and he said yes. He thinks she should be more alert and lively by Monday. I asked him what he would do if she wasn't; he said let's see how she is on Monday and then he can make a prognostication. I asked whether we should take another scan to see about swelling; he said not yet. He said her blood chem looks pretty good; her sugar is a little low and I could give her more juice.

I got Stel in the wheelchair and took her outside to watch Cindy in the pool. We came back to the room for dinner. Stel had right-side rigidity and was spacing out—she seemed to be somewhere else. When I asked her a couple of times where she was, she tried to respond, stuttering a lot. A new doctor came to evaluate Stel for physical therapy, which I had mentioned to Dr. R a couple of days ago. When she asked Stel a couple of questions about whether she had pain, she answered "yes" and "no." The doctor will make a ten-day schedule of exercises that Maribel will do. After ten days, the doctor will come back to see whether Stel needs different exercises. She said Stel's spasticity will come and go because a lot is going on in her head. Afterward, Stel got very rigid and seemed to be hallucinating a lot. She seemed so anxious. I held her and tried to calm her. I asked the nurse if she could have a sedative. Dr. Vasquez gave her a natural one. When the sedative kicked in, Stel went to sleep. (Stel tried to say something a few times late in the day, as she came out of her right-side "spells.")

Sat, May 13, 2000

Stel wasn't responsive and was sleepy all morning. When she had a right-side "spell," I hugged and kissed her. She said "Nobody…" Later, when I said "Stella," she said "yes" and looked at me. When I asked if she liked her lunch, she said "yes." After lunch she started to dose off, then opened her eyes and looked off to the right at the ceiling. Stel vomited beet juice twice when the nurses came to clean her up. When Dr. Perez, a psychiatrist, came in, I asked him if Stel's looking to the right could be a seizure. He said it could be and he would do a neurological exam. He checked her eyes, reflexes, ability to feel pain. He said the fact she could feel a pinch but nothing less showed the cortex wasn't functioning properly. Stel continued to sleep and sleep; when she was awake, she seemed to be having "spells." She spoke hardly at all today and wanted to sleep all the time.

Sun, May 14, 2000

When I gave Stel her medicines this morning, she clamped down on a pill with her teeth and I couldn't move it. Finally, she let it go, but I couldn't get her to swallow pills. During breakfast, she started swishing the tea in her mouth. She finally choked on it and spit it out. She was completely silent and oblivious to me. I started crying because I didn't see any change this morning and because I can't talk to her and can't get a response. I cried even harder when she was oblivious to my crying. When I stood in front of her and got her attention, she followed me with her eyes. I told her how hard it is not to talk to her. She seemed alert and trying to communicate with her eyes. Throughout the morning, she kept dozing and waking up. Later in the morning, she took her pills okay. She didn't seem to be having spells as much, maybe because she's so sleepy. I couldn't get her to say anything. I tried to get her to watch a movie, but she went to sleep. She seemed out of it when she woke up. I asked her if she's trying because I can't tell. She responded, "trying" (her only words today).

About 4:45 PM I got her up. She was like a sack of potatoes and I barely got her into the wheelchair. Her head lolled back and eyes rolled up and I thought she had a seizure. Then her eyes seemed okay and I straightened her up. She was leaning a little to the left but a pillow straightened her up (she hasn't had the leaning to left or right problem since we came down here). I took her to the dining room for dinner. She kept looking down all through dinner and after. But wonder of wonders, when I took her back to the room, I got her to look at "Superman" and she watched it intently. She continued to watch intently after I put her back in bed. Her eyes were bright and sparkling; she was looking at me and following me with her eyes. She watched TV until after 9 PM.

Mon, May 15, 2000

Stel seemed more alert when she woke up—perhaps a slight smile on her lips. But no words at all even though she looked on the verge of it. When I exercised her, her right side was tense and left hand was in a tight grip. Her left leg and foot were okay. When I asked her where she was because she seemed out of it, she tried to say something twice. She watched TV pretty intently until about 10 AM when she got sleepy. After she was cleaned up, she slept until lunch. I woke her up to eat, but she continued to be very sleepy. I said, "more pasta?" and she replied, "more pa...pa..." The nurse came in the room and asked me if a plate on the table was "su plato." Stel repeated, "su plato." Drs. C and T checked Stel; Dr. T said he did see any big changes. Stel slept through the checkup.

Around 2:00 PM, I woke Stel up to do exercises. She paid attention to me, but there were no words. Dr. Rubio said he can give her a preliminary vaccine tomorrow, which should make the immune system respond more quickly. He decided to increase the oxygen treatment to every two hours for twenty minutes. He's giving her more paladium. Stel will have a CT scan tomorrow. I got Stel up in the wheelchair. She stood pretty well. She sat up and looked at the TV for a while. Took her to the dining room for dinner. When I put her back to bed, she started watching the BBC news. As Maribel was doing her exercises, she said "okay," and Stel repeated "okay."

Tue, May 16, 2000

Took Stel for a CT scan today, to Notre Dame Hospital in Tijuana. Stel moved her head a few times because of right-side "spells" but otherwise did very well. She was pretty alert when we returned and she had lunch. Her eyes were bright and following me, but when I gave her the oxygen, she went to sleep and slept all afternoon. Just before dinner, Stel was more awake and alert and afterwards she watched the TV news. Dr. R came in and told me the CT scan showed a problem with "a little water in the ventricle," which is probably why Stel hasn't responded as he had anticipated. He thinks it's probably blocked by scar tissue and said he may be able to take care of this by increasing Rodakem, the diuretic he's been giving Stel. He said he's had this problem once before and that worked. If it works, it will do so in a few days. I'm upset about this and worried that the medication won't work. I remember reading about problems with hydrocephalus on the BT List. But I'm relieved that maybe this is the reason Stel hasn't shown more progress, because it's something that can be dealt with. While Maribel was exercising Stel, Stel moved her left foot several times. She was given the preliminary vaccine tonight. She spoke no words at all today.

Wed, May 17, 2000

Bill Blakley's grandmother came in to see Stel today. She talked to Stel, and I thought Stel might respond to her because she might remind Stel of her mother, but nothing happened. She was very sleepy for most of the day, barely awake when I was exercising her. Her left side was loose, the right side a little stiff. She started looking off in space and it was very hard to get her to focus on me; she wasn't trying to make any response at all. I was very worried and called Dr. C. I told him I'm very worried and wanted to talk to Dr. R. today. Dr. R. came in and told me he's going to increase the Rodakem and the aminos he's giving her. In 24-48 hours she may have some reaction from the vaccine. After that, I got Stel in the wheelchair. She was very limp and sleepy. We sat outside for about two hours. She had her head down all the time, even though she was awake. Bill B. helped me get her back to bed. When I tucked her in, I kissed her and told her how much I love her. She uttered a cry—of anguish it seemed—and looked at me for a long time. I felt so sad but so loving, and at least connected to her in a way I haven't for several days. I felt she was "here," in the moment. She went to sleep and when I woke her by kissing her, her eyes were alert; she was watching me and paying attention. I tried to get her to speak to me, to say Kate, but couldn't get a response. She dozed off with the oxygen, but then became alert and watched TV. She seemed a little flushed and sweaty and I wondered if that was a reaction to the vaccine. No words again today. It's wearing me down and I'm worrying that I should just take her and leave, but I hate to leave before she's had the real vaccine shot. It's been just a month since her last MRI; in another week or so I'm going to insist on another one. I'm terrified the tumor may be growing and causing these problems.

Thu, May 18, 2000

Stel woke up on her own, seemed more alert early, watching TV, but no words. Bill Blakley worked on Stel's feet again. She made several noises and was paying attention to him. When I asked her how she felt, she made another anguished sound. As I was exercising her legs, she moved her left foot and toes when I patted the inside of her thigh, as she did last night with Maribel. Don't know whether this is all reflex, but I don't think so. Bill's grandmother came in and talked to Stel again. She told her she's pretty and was astounded that Stel is sixty. She talked to Stel about her children. Stel looked at her intently, with a pleasant expression, but didn't try to speak. During and after lunch, Stel was staring at the ceiling. I talked to her and begged her to try to speak. She seemed to take it in, but she only made guttural sounds once or twice. She kept staring at the ceiling. It frightened me. Later, I got Stel up in the wheelchair. She was very limp. We went outside. The whole time, she sat with her head down, mostly sleeping. When she was awake, she seemed to be having right-side spells. After an hour, I put her back to bed, still very limp.

I met with Dr. R and told him I was very worried because Stel hasn't responded at all and is so sleepy and out of it much of the time. He said he would increase the Poly-MVA she's getting, as well as the Rodakem and growth hormone and would begin giving her Phosphotil Coline and Argenine—amino acids—as well as Hydragine—meant to reconnect brain cells. He feels the hydrocephalus is the problem. He said he had another case like this in 1987. The patient was slow to respond, but he kept increasing medications and finally she did. He thinks Stel will, too. He said he starts low on the meds so he can keep adding and increasing them. We talked about placement of a shunt, but he didn't think that was necessary now. It could be done in a hospital in San Diego. He agreed to schedule an MRI in San Diego next week. He gave me his beeper and home phone numbers so I can reach him when he's not here.

Stel was a little more awake after dinner, but she was having right-side problems. While Maribel was exercising her arms and legs, Stel said "no." After that, she watched TV news and a program about a train trip through Scotland.

Fri, May 19, 2000

Stel woke herself up. She seemed pretty alert and responsive when I kissed her. When I said "hi," she responded with a weak "hi." She watched TV, listened to the radio. She was relating to me with her eyes. I told her she needed to sign her name to a form the lawyer sent so he could retain an expert witness for the lawsuit and helped her write her name. I read Linda's letter to her. She seemed to take most of this in. She was alert through lunch, then slept more than an hour. Then I got her up; she was limp. As I put her in her wheelchair, she said "no." I took her outside. She had her head down but was awake most of the time. She looked over at me as I sat on the edge of the pool and watched intently for a few minutes. She also watched Cindy in the water a little bit. At the dinner table she had her head down. After dinner, Stel watched the Lehrer news program and then "Providence." I told Dr. R that Stel was more awake and alert today. He said let's just keep giving her the meds and see what happens. Steve called and said he's coming down tomorrow, which made me very happy.

Sat, May 20, 2000

Stel woke herself up about 7:15, but she wasn't responsive with her eyes this morning. She was having some right-side problems. She had trouble taking pills and they had to be crushed. She was so sleepy through lunch that she only ate a little bit and then wouldn't open her mouth. I managed to get some drinks and pills down her, but she was very sleepy. She was awake when Steve came in, but she didn't acknowledge him in any way and then went to sleep for a couple of hours. Steve and I talked; it was a great relief to me to have someone here with me. Later, I got her in the wheelchair and took her outside with Steve and me. She was sleeping in the chair and having right-side problems. I got dinner from the dining room and brought it outside. Stel ate soup and a little pasta and veggies but was too sleepy to finish. But after dinner, as I was telling Steve about Stel's documentary film project on Kambanellis and our research and writing about the Dodd family, Stel suddenly perked up and listened intently, looking at Steve. I was so happy. Before Steve left, we got Stel back to bed and then I told her I was going to sneak her a piece of lemon cake Steve had brought—like he used to bring to our house years ago—even though such sweets were forbidden on the hospital diet. Stel paid close attention and began to smile; then she looked right at Steve and laughed heartily. We both were very excited and felt like a million dollars. Steve said "yes, yes," and we encouraged her to say something, but she didn't. It was fantastic to hear her laugh so strongly! Afterwards, Stel was very sleepy and I had a hard time getting pills and Poly-MVA down her. She was so tired she wouldn't drink, but when I begged her to drink, she managed to do it. No words today.

Sun, May 21, 2000

Stel ate breakfast well and took her pills well, but she was very sleepy all morning. Her limbs were mostly flaccid. Steve came in late morning. As we talked, I noticed that Stel was listening, particularly when I talked about her friends in D.C. and giving them scarves Chris had designed. She looked very interested and smiled and then laughed again, looking at Steve. But she didn't speak. She was dozing off as Steve left, but she looked at him. After she slept for a couple of hours, I got her up and outside. She slept part of the time, but when I got in the swimming pool, she turned her head toward me and seemed to be watching me. We had dinner in the dining room and Stel helped eat her taco (she held it and I helped her get it to her mouth). While she seemed to be having a right-side spell, she was saying "baby, baby," apparently referring to a baby a visitor had brought with her. The woman brought the baby to show Stel and she looked intently at him. When I got her back in bed, she immediately went to sleep and slept all night without moving.

Mon, May 22, 2000

Stel was sleepy all morning. When Dr. C came in, I showed him a red spot on Stel's hip that I was afraid was a bedsore. I asked if they had bandages like those we had used for her heel. He said Dr. R has a special powder he uses and he will tell the nurse to get that for Stel. After lunch, I talked to Stel about how much I miss her, how much we have to do together. She was looking at me and seemed to be taking it in, but much of the time she was having right-side problems. She was sweaty. I got her up—she was limp—and took her outside. She sat with her head down. She was awake but seemed out of it. Her head was always down. Dr. R saw her. He said her head is down because of the pressure caused by the hydro-cephalus. He thought she should have more radiation, which could help open a path that is now blocked. I questioned him about this and told him I was reluc-tant to let her get more radiation. He urged that we try it again—in the same small doses; he believes it will help with the hydrocephalus. I finally agreed and she will have radiation tomorrow. I don't like doing it, but Dr. R persuaded me maybe it will help. I'm anxious to get the MRI this week because I'm so worried that Stel's sleepiness may indicate the tumor is growing. Dr. R also said Stel will get the vaccine tomorrow evening. He will have the nurse monitor her every hour after that. I'm relieved she can finally get the vaccine, which I hope will start to have a positive effect on her. After dinner, Stel was so sleepy I couldn't get her to drink her juice or take meds. She slept all evening. NO WORDS TODAY.

Tue, May 23, 2000

Stel was pretty alert when she woke up. She took all her pills and drank her juice well. When she made a noise like she was hurting, I asked her what was wrong and she said, "It's [unintelligible]…" She ate a good breakfast. After she ate, she got sleepy. When I tried to give her a pill and asked her if she swallowed it, she said "no." Her limbs were very flexible. In the midst of doing her exercises, I asked her where she was and she said something. At midday we went for a radia-tion session. When we got back, Stel ate her lunch with gusto. Then she went to sleep. Later in the afternoon, I got her up in the wheelchair in the room. She had her head down. I tried to get her to watch a movie, but she couldn't raise her head. I took her to the dining room for dinner. She ate well. When I put her back to bed, she immediately went to sleep. I tried to get her to take her meds, but she couldn't swallow them. I told Dr. C and he and Maribel tried to stimulate Stel to wake her up and tried to get the meds down her. Finally she was able to swallow them with some carrot juice. At 9:00 PM, Dr. V gave Stel the vaccine shot. Every hour after that until early morning, the nurse and I checked her temperature, pulse, blood pressure, and respiration. The only possible response to the vaccine that we measured was a slight increase in her respiration.

Wed, May 24, 2000

Stel ate her breakfast well, but she went back to sleep as soon as she had eaten. Her arms and legs were quite loose. She was mostly very sleepy or staring at the ceiling or into space, making me wonder if she's had a seizure. She was sleepier than yesterday. I had a long talk with Dr. C. He said Martha Baker didn't respond that fast; it was up and down. Then one day she just clicked. Stel's tumor is smaller than Martha's but more central and is blocking the ventricles. All they need is a little opening to get the medicine through. The vaccine shot was very strong, he said, and it might make her sleepy. While he was checking her, she made a noise and rolled her eyes to the ceiling. Took her to another radiation session. Afterward, she ate a good lunch and then went to sleep. Dr. R came in and checked her; he said her neck was looser and this indicated less pressure in the brain. Her respiration was at 24, which indicated a reaction to the vaccine, he said. After dinner, Maribel did her exercises and thought Stel's limbs were looser. NO WORDS.

Thu, May 25, 2000

Took Stel to radiation again. She was awake the whole time and when we came back, she ate every bite of her lunch. She wasn't able to take pills or other meds very well today. I talked to her, implored her, but she wasn't reachable. I got Stel up in the afternoon. She was holding her head up higher than she has in days and was quite alert. Dr. R said this is a good sign that pressure is alleviating. He said he will give her a second vaccine shot tomorrow. Stel ate dinner in the dining room. She was alert. Jake [a young patient] came to introduce himself and Stel paid attention to him. She ate well but as time wore on, she got more tired and her head kept dropping, but she was wide awake. When I put her to bed, she rolled her eyes up to the ceiling and I had a hard time getting her to look at me. Stel was more awake today than yesterday. NO WORDS AGAIN.

Fri, May 26, 2000

We took Stel to San Diego for an MRI. When I wheeled her out to the van, she had her head up and was looking straight ahead. They lifted her onto a reclining chair in the van. Because of the delay in getting across the border, we were half an hour late and so we had to wait another hour-and-a-half before they could work her in for the scan. She slept during that time. I got a copy of the scan and was very relieved to see that the tumor looks about the same size as it did on the April MRI. I was so afraid it was growing. Stel was too sleepy to eat lunch when we got back. As I was exercising her, I said, "You're sleepy, sleepy, sleepy," and she repeated that. That evening, when Maribel was exercising Stel, she asked Stel to give her her hand and Stel did! Maribel was talking to her about how lonely I am when Stel doesn't talk and Stel started laughing. Then she kissed Maribel's hand! Later, Judy came in and Stel looked at her with a little smile. She paid attention to Dr. C when he gave her her vaccine shot. She was definitely more alert. We monitored her vital signs every hour. Her blood pressure and temperature went up.

Sat, May 27, 2000

Stel ate a good breakfast and lunch, but was very sleepy. About 4:00 PM I got her up. In the wheelchair, she was looking off in space, then she started looking down. Her right side was rigid. I tried to get her to watch TV, but she kept looking off. It was easier to raise her head than other days, but when it wasn't supported, it was mostly down. Outside, her eyes were open, but she wasn't here. She was having right-side problems, leaning forward, looking down. During dinner, her head was down the whole time. When I put her back to bed and turned her on her side to avoid bed sores, she went to sleep immediately. Dr. C came in and I told him it had been a bad day. He said she's responding a little and he thinks she will click one day. NO WORDS TODAY.

Sun, May 28, 2000

Stel was sleepy all morning and not able to take her meds. When I exercised her, her left side was really flaccid—it worries me. Her right side was flexible but Stel indicated pain when I flexed her right arm. She slept and slept. Just before noon I put on Alan Parsons music and danced a little. She was awake and seemed to pay some attention. She ate a good lunch and I managed to get Depakote down her and a glass of grape juice with MVA, etc. I couldn't get other pills down. I got her up about 4:30. She couldn't stand up. I barely got her in the chair. She held her head mostly up. At dinner, Stel held her taco part of the time. She ate everything. I tried to get her to watch TV, but she kept her head down. I talked to her about how upset I am, how she doesn't seem to care whether I'm here, that there's no special connection. She seemed to listen and made some noises but she didn't say anything, even when I cried. When I put her back to bed, she watched a little TV but then quickly went to sleep. As I was turning her later, she tried to say something three times, as if she was in some discomfort.

Mon, May 29, 2000

Stel was pretty much awake this morning. She watched some TV. I turned her and doctored her sores. (Dr. R's powder seems quite effective.) Her limbs were pretty loose. As I was moving her legs, I told Stel we were doing the bicycle and she became very alert and paid attention to me. At 9:50 AM she watched a cooking show on TV very steadily. Drs. Smith and Tapia came in to check Stel. Dr. T wanted to see the MRI. When I cleaned Stel's nose and showed her gigantic boogers, she laughed. Took her for another radiation session. When we got back, she ate well, then dozed off. Later, I got Stel up and took her outside. She had some right-side problems. She was mainly awake, looking down, but I could raise her head with some effort. She ate in the dining room. When I put her back to bed, I held her while she stood; she straightened her knee once and stood with difficulty for a couple of minutes. While Maribel was exercising her, Stel laughed and continued smiling slightly at her. Dr. C came in and talked to her and she was alert. Cathy called in the evening and I put Stel on the phone; she listened intently and said "yes." When Cathy said good bye, a slight smile crossed Stel's lips. I asked her if she was glad to talk to Cathy and she faintly said "yes." She was alert and watched TV—an animal story—until 8:30 PM Stel was more awake for more time today and alert late.

Tue, May 30, 2000

Stel was awake early. She indicated pain and I found her leg wedged against the bed railing. It obviously had been there for hours because there was a dent in her leg. She mostly watched TV until 10:30 AM and was still awake when I gave her oxygen. Before this, Drs. Smith and Tapia came in. Dr. Smith said Stel seemed more alert than yesterday. Stel's limbs were flexible; her left limbs were quite limp, which worries me. Another radiation session today—thank god Dr. R said tomorrow would be the last. He said he would give her another vaccine shot tomorrow. He was encouraged by the fact that she had some response to the last shot. He told me to hang in there. Stel slept a lot in the afternoon. In between dozing off, she watched some of the BBC news. When Maribel came, we got Stel up and tried to have her stand, but she was too limp. Maribel did exercises with her in the wheelchair. Stel was awake but looking off in space, not here. We both tried to get her attention. Finally, I hugged her and asked her to come back to be with us. She looked at me and connected, then looked at Maribel. For a few moments we were able to connect with her. I asked her to stand with us and she did—even straightened her legs once or twice! She stood maybe two minutes. Then we put her in bed and she went to sleep about 8:00 PM. NO WORDS TODAY.

Wed, May 31, 2000

Stel was very sleepy and unresponsive this morning, but when Drs. Smith and Tapia came in later, they thought she was more alert, following them with her eyes, but I told them this is nothing new. Took her to her tenth and last radiation session today. Dr. R said the MRI report from San Diego indicated the tumor is slightly smaller. Also, the fluid problem is now only in the front right side. He thinks we should taper down anti-seizure meds so she will be more awake. He'll talk to me further tomorrow about the MRI report. I got a copy of the report and saw that the measurements in it were about 1.3 cm smaller than the measurements in the April report. I was so happy and told Stel the tumor was definitely smaller. I talked to her for some time about how good this is and how it indicates we're going in the right direction. Stel looked at me and listened intently even though she said nothing. Later, Dr. C came in and said Stel's Tegretol level from several days ago was very high. This could explain some of her sleepiness and lethargy. They will proceed to reduce anti-seizure meds. While Maribel was exercising Stel in the evening, Stel was looking off in space despite M's efforts to get her to engage. But when Imelda (the evening nurse) came in and she and M talked and laughed, Stel started smiling widely. She looked at both of them and followed Imelda with her eyes. She was quite engaged. We got her to stand up and she stood very well—her feet flat and straightening her knees once—knees straight for probably four minutes. When we put her back to bed and clapped and cheered for her, she had a slight smile on her face and her eyes were bright. She looked proud! Maribel commented again on how pretty Stel is and asked me to show Imelda her photo. Imelda called her "muy bonita." As soon as we got her settled, Stel went to sleep about 7:00 PM. At 8:45 PM. they gave her a third vaccine shot. No words again.

Thu, June 1, 2000

BIG DAY!! Stel was alert, smiling all afternoon! In the morning, she was pretty groggy. I talked to her but got no response and I was very upset. Dr. Smith came in in late morning and said Stel's Tegretol level was too high, making her sleepy and lethargic. She would become more alert when level was reduced, but Tegretol stays in the system several weeks and it's hard to reduce. Patience is necessary. I was feeling very low after lunch as I turned Stel and was going to let her sleep. But I saw she was very alert and noticing people as they walked by outside the window. She seemed so with it that I stayed talking to her about how she's going to beat this and what we're going to do. She was very engaged and had a pleasant look on her face. I kissed her and she kissed and kissed back. Then she smiled and laughed. I played music for over an hour and sang and danced at her bedside, holding her hands. She watched and listened and seemed to be fully engaged and wide awake—much more so than in previous days. I FELT JOYFUL—LIKE WE HAD TURNED A CORNER.

In mid-afternoon, I got her up and took her outside. She stood up well for the transfer. Outside, at first she paid attention to people and looked up at them with her eyes wide open. She looked at Delfina [a nurse] and smiled. Elena [the mother of another patient] showed Stel her cross-stitching and Stel seemed to be interested at first. Then she started having right-side problems and started shaking, with her head down. But she was wide awake, not dozing at all. She kept looking up at me with wide eyes, fully engaged. When Dr. R came, I told him how alert she had been. He said phasing down the meds would make her more alert and he thinks by Monday she'll probably be talking. He will give her another vaccine shot on Monday and she'll get a CT scan on Thursday. At dinner in the dining room, Stel looked down the whole time and had continuous right-side spells, leaning abruptly forward and looking down as if she was seeing something. She was shaking a lot and sweating. After she was back in bed, she looked at Lilly [a nurse] and smiled. She did the same thing when Delfina came in to change her IV. She watched the BBC news intently. While Maribel was exercising her, Stel looked at her and smiled and laughed several times, as she did when Delfina came in again. Both M and D told her how beautiful she is and Maribel said she looks like a baby (which she does). Stel had a pleasant look on her face the whole time.

Fri, June 2, 2000
ANOTHER RED LETTER DAY!!

Stel was awake and alert early. She followed the nurses and me with her eyes. She was clearly here. As I was giving her breakfast, I asked her if she liked the watermelon. She said "yes." She was paying attention to everything and everyone today. Judy came in the room and Stel looked at her and smiled and laughed; when Judy asked her if she was feeling better, she answered "yes" and looked like she was going to say more. Dr. S came in and was amazed to see how alert she was; she said Stel was so much better. Stel looked at her and laughed. Before lunch, I put the Steve Martin movie, "Bowfinger" on and Stel watched it with me for twenty minutes or so. SHE LAUGHED IN THE APPROPRIATE PLACES 2-3 TIMES. When I turned it off so she could have lunch, I asked her if she liked the movie and she said "yes." I said "Steve Martin is a good writer," and she answered emphatically, "Yes, he is." After lunch, I asked Stel if she had enjoyed it and she responded "yes." When I put the movie back on, Stel laughed at one funny part. Then she seemed to get tired, so I turned it off; but she didn't go to sleep. I played music and she kept looking at me intensely. I asked her a question and she said "yes." I kissed her and she kissed and kissed back in a very sexy way.

I said, "you little devil," and she laughed. When I asked her how she felt, she said, "pretty good." I asked her if she felt tired and she said, "no." She also responded "no" when I asked her if she wanted some grapes. Delfina came in and talked to Stel and Stel laughed.

I got Stel up and took her outside. She laughed when Bertha [the receptionist] talked to her. I asked her if she liked being outside and she said, "yes." When Dr. R came, I told him that Stel had been extremely alert and responsive today and I was very encouraged. She spoke to the doctor for the first time, responding "very good" when he asked her how she felt. He said he thinks her right-side problems will become less in the next few days. (She didn't have as severe a problem today as yesterday, but enough that she had her head down most of the time. But when called, she would look up with big wide eyes. At dinner, she did look around the table a little bit.) Back in the room, Maribel and I tried to have Stel stand but she couldn't do it very well. When we put her to bed like a sack of potatoes, Stel laughed. Later, as I was turning her over, I muttered to myself, "Protection brigade for derrieres," and Stel laughed. I said, "I've said a lot of crazy things trying to get you to laugh." SHE STUTTERED, "THAT WAS VERY FUNNY." I told her I saw a difference in her starting yesterday when her eyes followed different things and asked if she felt the difference. She said "no." I asked if she knew she was beautiful and she said "no." (It's remarkable how many people say Stel is beautiful.)

Sat, June 3, 2000

Stel was awake early and was responsive with her eyes. When Myra came in, Stel watched her. Myra said "hi" and told Stel her name. Stel said, "Hi, My…"—stuttering the name. Myra asked Stel her name but Stel didn't respond. Her feet and arms had more tone today than for some time; her legs were flexible. Lilly tried to get Stel to speak or smile, but she didn't, although she watched Lilly alertly. She watched intently when Martha Stewart was cooking on TV. When I kissed Stel, she gave me long kisses back even though her chin was tremoring a lot. In the afternoon, I danced, holding her hands; she looked out the door behind me at a little boy who was crying. I said, "he's sure screaming," and Stel laughed. I got her up at 4:30. She stood up strongly. Her head was mostly up at first. As we waited out front for dinner, her head drooped more and she didn't pay attention to anyone. Her head was down throughout dinner. After dinner, as Maribel worked with Stel, Stel looked at her and laughed. We had Stel stand up for 2-3 minutes. She did pretty well—straightened herself once. In bed, she moved her right leg herself while Maribel was exercising her. Stel wasn't as "here" today as yesterday, but when I tried to engage her, I usually could get eye contact. Few words today.

Sun, June 4, 2000

Stel was alert early, her eyes were responsive, following me, but no words. Adrianna [a nurse] tried to get her to talk, but she didn't. Stel ate her watermelon and eggs with my help. She was able to initiate putting bites in her mouth. I asked her if she liked the eggs and she said, "yes." She wasn't paying much attention to the nurses this morning, but she was communicating with her eyes frequently. No smiles. Cathy called and as I was telling her that Stel was slightly smiling when Cathy talked to her, Stel laughed. She stood up strongly when I transferred her to the wheelchair, and she sat with her head up for ten minutes or so. Then, progressively, it dropped lower. She looked up when Shirley [the mother of another patient] talked to her. During lunch her head was up more than usual and I did get her to look around a couple of times. Outside, she sat with her head way down and had right-side spells. She sat up in the chair more than four hours. After I put her back in bed, I asked Stel if she was awake and she said, weakly, "yes." During and after dinner, Stel was quite alert. She paid attention to Delfina when she spoke to her. She watched a movie about Vietnam and I WAS AMAZED WHEN WE LAUGHED AT THE SAME MOMENT. STEL WATCHED ALL OF THE MOVIE, THEN WATCHED THE END OF "CRADLE WILL ROCK," AND THEN ANOTHER MOVIE. She dozed off about 9:00 PM. Few words today.

Mon, June 5, 2000

Stel was shaking a lot this morning; very bad tremors in both arms and hands and chin. She had a couple of severe right-side contractions—she pulled her knee way up and said "oh." When I exercised her, there were a lot of tremors and tone in all limbs. I was so discouraged. Despite this, though, she was still more awake and alert later and watched TV. Dr. Tapia checked her arms and legs; he thinks she's getting better—more alert, responding more to sensations like tweaking her toes. She dozed off just before lunch, but woke up and responded strongly when I kissed her. I WAS STANDING BY THE BED, BLOCKING HER VIEW OF THE TV AND SHE WAS LOOKING AT ME BUT LAUGHING AT THE JOKES (WHICH WERE FUNNY) IN A CAROL BURNETT SKIT!! AS I WAS GIVING HER LUNCH, SHE LAUGHED AT MORE JOKES SHE HEARD!!

Dr. R said he would give her another vaccine shot tonight. He believes that by next week she'll be doing better. It's a matter of time. She's responding. The tremors will get better as her brain does. At 4:15 PM I got Stel up. She stood well. While we were waiting for dinner in the dining room, Maribel talked to Stel and Stel looked at her and laughed. She paid attention to both Maribel and Bertha when they spoke to her. At dinner, she ate some of her food with my help, as she did at breakfast. Back in the room, Stel sat almost all the time with her head down, but she could look up when motivated. When I kissed her, she kissed back. Maribel and I tried to get Stel to stand up with the walker. She stood up strongly, but her left foot kept turning. M tried to get Stel to speak, but she didn't, even though she looked at M intently. But when M told Stel that she (Maribel) was talking like a parrot to Stel, Stel laughed. Stel got her fourth vaccine shot at 9:30 PM When I turned her, I asked if she was comfortable. She said, "yes." Adrianna then talked to her and Stel laughed. Just over an hour after the shot, Stel had a major seizure. Shortly after that, I realized her respiration was very low. Dr. C gave her oxygen and Decadron and other medications and she gradually breathed easier. I was beside myself!

Tue, June 6, 2000

Stel was awake early. She seemed able to focus, took her meds okay and drank her juice. She was still breathing very slowly—10—but the oxygen saturation was okay. She ate a good breakfast, but she was very sleepy. She was out of it a lot of the time. Dr. R said she had the seizure because the vaccine shot was too powerful. For the next one on Friday he'll drop the number of cells back to 80,000. She probably was breathing slowly, he said, because of the message to the motor area after the cells attacked the tumor. But it wasn't a problem because she was breathing deeply and her oxygen saturation was okay. After the CT scan results on Thursday, we'll talk about how much longer he thinks we should be here. I told him we had to leave soon.

Later in the day I got Stel up. She stood very strongly with her feet flat. She sat up better than she has; her head was down but not too far. M and I had Stel stand up with the walker four times. She couldn't get her upper body straight, but her left foot was flat on the floor. When M worked with her in bed, Stel was able to hold her left leg with knee bent on the bed. But she was off in space and didn't smile or laugh at M even though she looked at her several times. NO WORDS; NO LAUGHS TODAY.

Wed, June 7, 2000

After breakfast, I talked to Stel about being involved in her exercise and how she doesn't want to be an invalid. She was listening and made a cry. Dr. Smith came in and talked to Stel. She looked at her but said nothing. Stel was sleeping and sleeping today. She couldn't even finish eating. Back to square one. Chris called and when Stel heard him, she uttered a faint, "yes." At 4:00 PM, I got her up and we sat outside. Her head was down. She wasn't here and had some right-side spells. After dinner, we tried to have Stel stand, but she couldn't do it very well. When we put her back to bed, the nurses changed her catheter. After that, she was more awake. When Dr. Vasquez came in, she was eating an apple and quite alert. She winced when he gave her shots. He said she was much more alert than he had seen her.

Thu, June 8, 2000

Took Stel for CT scan. It went fine. She stayed still. She was awake, looking at ambulance men and the machine operator. When we got back, she was sleepy and went to sleep after lunch. I woke her up at 2:30, played music and talked to her. She was alert, looking at me, but not speaking or smiling. I got her out of bed at 3:30. She stood pretty well. In the wheelchair, she was looking down. Dr. R said to hold her head up and massage her neck once a day. Told me he would get CT scan results later and would talk to me tomorrow about everything. Stel slept most of day and evening.

Fri, June 9, 2000

At 4:00 AM I woke up and checked on Stel. I was frightened when I saw blood on her pillow, but when I checked, I saw the blood was coming from a sore on the back of her left ear. I called the nurse who took care of it. Later in the morning, when Stel was being cleaned up, she vomited. She slept most of morning. Dr. R told me the CT scan report says tumor shrank by almost half. I was startled by this and wanted to believe it but said I couldn't really put my trust in a CT scan. I'd have to see it on an MRI. I told him I wasn't seeing any clinical evidence of such shrinkage. He said he thought this was because of the fluid on the brain and he would increase Rodakem and Hydragine. I told him we have to go home next week and have her surgeon deal with it if necessary. He said that would be okay; we could return in a few weeks for follow-up. Before we leave, he will give Stel three more vaccine shots; he's giving her so many because of the hydrocephalus problem. Re the bleeding ear, he said he thought that was caused by the diaper they put around her head to hold the cabbage poultice every night. It rubbed against the ear. Dr. R said he wouldn't give Stel a vaccine shot tonight because of the late effect of the previous shot (vomiting). He thought her sleepiness is probably a delayed reaction to the last shot, too. He'll give her an anti-emetic. Maribel exercised Stel's legs, but she was so sleepy she couldn't open her eyes. NO WORDS TODAY.

Sat, June 10, 2000

After I gave Stel her juice, I told her I would get her breakfast, "okay?". She answered, "okay." Later, I said something else to her and she started to respond, "The…" She was pretty alert during breakfast. After breakfast, she got sleepy again. For lunch, she ate all of her soup and a little fish but was too sleepy to finish. She slept most of the afternoon. I got her up at 3:30. She stood pretty well, but sat in the chair with her head way down the whole time. After dinner in the dining room, I put her back to bed. She couldn't stand up well. She slept all evening.

Sun June 11, 2000

Stel was sleeping most of the morning and afternoon. I got her up at 4:00 PM. She stood fairly well. Sitting, her head was down but not as much as yesterday. We ate outside. I put her back to bed at 6:00. She was having right-side spells and looking off in space most of the time. When I kissed her, she kissed back several times. She was more alert in the evening—watching a little TV and looking at me. She was also having right-side problems. When Dr. Perez came to give her shots, he asked if she remembered him; she said, "yes." Then he asked how she was and she responded, "well"—faintly. He said he thought she looks and seems much better.

Mon, June 12, 2000

Stel was pretty alert, noticing people moving outside the door, until after 10:00 AM. Then she dozed off and on into the afternoon. I got her up at 4:00. Dr. R told me he wouldn't give her a vaccine shot tonight but would wait to see how she is in the next days. Tomorrow, he will make a home plan so I can get together everything I need to take home by Friday. I put Stel to bed at 6:00 because I couldn't stand to see her sitting with her head down. AS MARIBEL WAS EXERCISING HER, M TOLD STEL SHE'S BEAUTIFUL AND STEL SMILED. WHEN MARIBEL ASKED STEL IF SHE ATE WELL, STEL SAID, "YES."

MARIBEL EXCLAIMED, "YOU'RE WONDERFUL," AND STEL LAUGHED. LATER, STEL SMILED AT MARIBEL. WHEN DELFINA CAME IN, SHE SPOKE TO STEL, SAYING HOW WONDERFUL SHE LOOKED AND STEL SMILED. LATER, I KISSED HER AND SHE KISSED BACK FOR A LONG TIME. THIS HAPPENED TWICE. I TOLD HER SHE'S VERY SEXY AND SHE LAUGHED. Dr. C. showed me how to give a shot with the small needle and I gave Stel her shot this evening. SHE WAS MUCH MORE ALERT TONIGHT, LOOKING AT ME AND AT THE TV UNTIL 9:30 PM.

Tue, June 13, 2000

Stel was alert in the morning but having a lot of right-side problems. After lunch, she went to sleep. At 3:00 I woke her up and did exercises with her. At 4:00, I got her up. She sat with her head down, but not as much as yesterday. We sat outside until dinner. Dr. R said he will give her a vaccine shot tomorrow night. He will explain the home program to me on Thursday. We can come back in six weeks for a follow-up. He believes her right-side rigidity, sleepiness, not talking is mostly because of the pressure in her head from fluid. After dinner, Maribel and I had Stel stand up twice. Her feet were flat on the floor. When she was in bed, she was paying attention to M but didn't smile or speak. I kissed her and she kissed back. She was awake until 10:00 and watched intently a documentary on "Four Little Girls," the black children killed in the bombing in Birmingham. NO WORDS TODAY.

Wed, June 14, 2000

When I was giving Stel her breakfast, I asked if she liked the potatoes and she said, "yes." She was very sleepy today and slept a lot of the time. I got her up at 3:30. She sat with her head down the whole time. After dinner, I put her back to bed and she immediately went to sleep. When Maribel exercised Stel's legs and arms, she couldn't get Stel to laugh or speak. She was very impassive and sleepy. Stel got her fifth vaccine shot tonight. IT WAS A VERY DISCOURAGING DAY.

Thu, June 15, 2000

Stel was sleepy this morning (she had been awakened every hour during the night to check her vital signs—her temperature and pulse went up slightly for a couple of hours). When she was awake, she seemed alert, noticing what's happening outside the door. Drs. S and T came in to see her. Dr. T thinks her lack of functioning is due both to hydrocephalus and radiation swelling. It will take about six weeks for the swelling to go down. She will be intermittently more and less alert. At lunch, as Stel was eating her soup, she started trying to vomit. The doctor gave her an anti-nausea shot, which made her sleepy and she slept most of the afternoon. I got her up at 4:30 and she sat with her head up higher than yesterday; but during dinner, her head was down a lot. Dr. R said her nausea was related to the vaccine shot. After dinner, Maribel and I got Stel to stand up twice. She did pretty well with her feet and knees, but her head was down and her body bent. M tried to get Stel to smile or speak but wasn't able to do so. After we put her back to bed, I kissed her and she gave me good kisses back. This was the only good moment today. I broke down in the evening. I'm so disappointed, frightened, lonely. Will Stella ever come back? ANOTHER DISCOURAGING DAY. NO WORDS. I checked with Adrianna and Dr. P and I think Stel may be getting more Decadron than she should be. MUST TALK TO DR. RUBIO ABOUT THIS.

Fri, June 16, 2000

Stel was awake most of the morning but not very responsive. While I was exercising her, I talked to her about trying to help, and I think she did keep her left leg straight for a short time. She didn't do it with the right. At lunch she was so sleepy she didn't finish eating and she slept most of the afternoon. LATER, I KISSED HER AND SHE KISSED AND KISSED BACK. It made me feel much better. I told her this, that it is our one way of communicating. It helps me to know she still loves me. IN THE EVENING WHEN M WAS EXERCISING STEL, SHE SANG "STELLA BELLA" TO STEL AND STEL LAUGHED. M ASKED STEL TO GIVE HER HER RIGHT HAND AND STEL MADE THAT EFFORT! STEL ALSO BENT HER RIGHT KNEE AND MOVED HER LEG. Afterward, she was pretty alert, watching TV news regarding Putin and the arrest of a publisher. BETTER DAY!

Sat, June 17, 2000

Stel was alert for a good part of the morning, but after lunch she was so sleepy I could hardly get her to take pills or drink juice. She slept until 4:00 when I got her up. Initially, her head wasn't way down, but progressively it sank lower. She was looking off in space all the time and hardly looked at me today. After dinner, M and I had her stand twice, but she was turning her left foot. M tried to get Stel to respond, but she either looked off in space or slept. THIS WAS ONE OF THE WORST DAYS. NO SMILES, NO WORDS, NO CONNECTION.

Sun, Jun 18, 2000

Stel was pretty sleepy in morning and afternoon. I got her up at 11:30. She was very limp. Her head was way down. We had lunch in the dining room. Steve came so I could give him some things to take back with him to ship to me. He will meet us at the airport tomorrow. Stel didn't engage with him at all, but when he left, she looked at him. She watched a TV movie until 8:00 p.m. WHEN I TUCKED HER IN, SHE KISSED ME PASSIONATELY. Tomorrow we go home so Dr. Neiman can deal with the hydrocephalus, which I hope will help Stel a lot and then we'll see how the vaccine is working.

End of Journal

Fri Jun 23 2000 8:16 AM

Steve, Just wanted to let you know that we got home okay. Getting Stel in and out of the car at 11-12 at night after a long, tiring day wasn't easy, but with the help of friends, we managed. I talked to her surgeon the next day and we'll be seeing her this coming week. We'll have an MRI done on Tuesday and will see her the same day. I'll let you know what she recommends. Stel has mostly been sleeping since we've been home and she hasn't tried to say anything now for well over a week. But she's still "here" at times and watched some TV last night. Unfortunately, she's so weak physically now that I'm having a very hard time getting her up from bed and back into bed by myself. It's a real problem. I've managed so far, but it takes far more energy by both of us than I'd like. It's a problem I don't have an answer to at the moment. Next week some of the volunteers we had previously will be coming in for a few hours on several days, and that will be of some help, but not as much as I need.

I've learned that there's one thing I just can't do—I can't give Stel shots with the larger needle. I just can't plunge the thing into her. I can deal, reluctantly, with the small needle. I've got a call in to Dr. Rubio to talk to him about it and find out what oral glandular formula he mentioned that I could give her. Also, I'm going to check with some people to see if there's a nurse or paramedic or someone around who might be willing to give Stel at least some of the shots for a reasonable fee. I wish I could find someone because I know the shots are very important.

Thanks again for your concern and help through these past very difficult weeks. Your visits and phone calls were lifesavers for me. And, of course, having your help at the airport was invaluable, not to mention having your assistance in shipping the excess back. Kay

Thu June 29 2000 5:21 AM

Dr. [Steven] Brem: Because I've seen such wonderful reports about you on the Brain Tumor List, I'm writing you regarding my partner, Stella Sandris, who was diagnosed with a GBM in May '99. I'd like to send some recent scans to you for an opinion. All of Stella's MRIs since late December have shown a stable situation, but she has not done well clinically. For several months she has not been able to do anything for herself and she's progressively talked less and less.

Currently, she's unable to hold her head up when she sits in the wheelchair (this has been going on for about six weeks). She's also stopped trying to talk completely. (This has been the case for about two weeks.) And she's sleeping a lot. (For the past six weeks or so.) One doctor believes the problem is fluid trapped on the brain. A late May MRI report refers to a "mild increase in generalized ventriculomegaly." However, based on an MRI done this week, Stella's surgeon said that she doesn't think the fluid problem is significant and wouldn't want to shunt Stella because of it. She said the only explanation she could give for why Stella isn't able to hold her head up, isn't talking, and is sleeping so much is that there are extensive "white matter changes" shown on the MRI. From what I could gather, she believes these changes are probably permanent and that Stella will not get any better.

The June 27th MRI report speaks of "persistent moderate ventriculomegaly." It further refers to "extensive and confluent increased inversion recovery and T2 signal involving virtually all of the white matter bilaterally, a finding which is most likely due to radiation treatment although progressive multifocal leukoencephalopathy cannot be excluded. These white matter findings are unchanged from the previous examination." The MRI report from the previous examination on April 17th (done at the same place but read by a different radiologist) did not say anything about white matter changes. It spoke only of "increased associated edema now involving almost the entire periventricular white matter at and above the level of the lateral ventricles." (Stella was sleeping a good bit at that time, too, and as a result of this report, we increased her steroid dose and she became more alert.) The June 27th report does note that "There is a considerable amount of associated surrounding edema which is difficult to discriminate from the extensive white matter change." From having looked at these scans over the past year or so, it certainly appears to me what is referred to as white matter change looks identical to what is called swelling on other scans.

I'm very confused and want to get some other opinions about this. Would it be possible to send the scans to you for a reading? Also, if you think white matter changes are a significant factor here, can you tell me what that portends for the future and for Stella's regaining any of her functions? Finally, would you think an MRSpectroscopy would help to sort things out better? I'm sorry for such a long message and look forward to hearing from you. Many thanks, Kay Loveland

NOTE: I came back from Mexico believing that many of Stel's problems were probably caused by hydrocephalus which could probably be rectified by the placement of a shunt by her neurosurgeon. When her surgeon told me she thought Stel's problems stemmed not from hydrocephalus but from "extensive white matter changes" that were the result of radiation treatment, I was completely non-plussed. It was one of those times when I felt that I had been side-swiped.

Section 3. The Last Five Months

Mon Jul 03 2000 7:34 AM

Margaret, The problems your daughter is having sound similar to Stel's problems. The tumor has been stable since the end of December, but she has functioned less and less well. Recent scans have shown a lot of enhancement throughout the brain which one radiologist interpreted as extensive swelling back in April and now, this past week, another—and Stel's surgeon—interpret as "white matter changes" that are probably permanent and could be scar tissue, dead tissue, and/or disease, all resulting from prior radiation, and possibly chemotherapy. This is the first time I've ever had anyone mention white matter changes—or brain disease from radiation and chemo—to me, and no radiologist or doctor before now has referred to it as a problem. Her Decadron dose is being boosted up from 12, probably to 24, to see if it helps her alertness, etc., which would indicate that we're dealing mostly with swelling (I HOPE). (There's also a possibility that mild hydrocephalus is causing some problems.) No one has told me why there would be so much swelling if the tumor is stable. However, I am getting scans out to several doctors in the next few days for further opinions and I'm going to ask if they don't tell.

Re improving functionality, a friend just told me last night about an article she had found in the Journal of Clinical Oncology on a study of a drug called methylphenidate [I didn't realize then that this is Ritalin], which apparently improves cognition, mood and functionality of brain tumor patients. It caused no increase in seizures and made it possible for some patients to decrease their Decadron dose. I'm e-mailing the researcher at MD Anderson this morning and am going to follow up on this aggressively. I've got to find something to help Stel. Also, re substitutes for Decadron, my friend also told me about a study of hCRF. Results of a Phase 1 study over two years ago apparently showed that it might be a good alternative to steroids for controlling edema. I'm following up on this as well. I'll let you know what I find out. All the best, Kay

Mon Jul 03 2000 7:59 AM

Dr. [Christina] Meyers: A friend of mine has advised me of an article in the Journal of Clinical Oncology in July 1998 regarding a study you did of 30 patients that showed functional improvement with the use of methylphenidate. I would like to find out more about this as soon as possible. I am caring for a brain tumor patient whose MRIs have been stable since December, but she has not functioned well during this time. Motivation, in particular, is a problem, as is incontinence and lack of ability to communicate. Is it possible to get methylphenidate prescribed for her? I will very much appreciate hearing from you as soon as possible about the current status of this drug and any further studies that have been, or are being, done. Thanks, Kay Loveland

Mon Jul 03 2000 9:57 AM

Dear Kay Loveland, I would be happy to send you a reprint of the article if you would provide your address. Currently we are proposing a placebo controlled randomized trial of Ritalin that the American College of Surgeons Oncology Group will sponsor, and we are also looking at trials of a new sustained release methylphenidate and new agents such as modafinil. Stimulant therapy really appears to have great benefit in brain tumor patients, as well as those with cancer-related fatigue. Dr. Christina Meyers

Mon Jul 03 2000 11:00 PM

Dear Dr. Meyers: Thank you for your reply. I am interested in whether it would be possible for my partner's oncologist to prescribe methylphenidate for her. It's not clear to me from your reply whether that is possible or not. If you prefer to deal directly with the oncologist, I can ask her to contact you.

I'm interested to know about your Ritalin study. Stella took a little Ritalin a few months ago—5 mg—and for the first 3-4 days, she was really lively and almost herself. Then it seemed to dissipate. Many thanks, Kay Loveland

Tue Jul 04 2000 8:33 AM

Dear Friends, Since today is Stel's birthday, it seems an appropriate time to send you an update. As some of you know, we returned from Mexico a couple of weeks ago (many thanks to those of you who called and wrote during the seven weeks we were down there). Unfortunately, as some of you also know, Stel didn't respond to the vaccine and other treatment in the dramatic way other brain tumor patients (two of whom I met there at the hospital) have. We all expected her to start functioning better within a matter of weeks, but it never happened. There were several days when she was very lively, trying to talk a good bit, laughing (even at funny lines in movies and TV shows) and we thought she was off and running, but they didn't last, and there were many more days when she was very sleepy and uncommunicative. Needless to say, it was a nerve-wracking time for me.

About two weeks after we got there, we did a CT scan which indicated that there was a problem with fluid drainage on Stel's brain. An MRI two weeks after that and another CT scan in early June continued to show a problem with this—not severe, but enough to make the doctors there believe that hydrocephalus was interfering with Stel's ability to respond to the treatment. The doctor tried to resolve the problem non-invasively, but by mid-June it seemed clear that this wasn't working. So we came back to the States on June 19th, ready to see Stel's surgeon and talk about surgical means of taking care of it. We had an MRI last week and saw the surgeon. Much to my surprise, she said she didn't think the fluid problem was significant enough to cause Stel to be so sleepy and uncommunicative and to have difficulties holding her head up when she sits in the wheelchair, and the surgeon wouldn't advise putting a shunt in for drainage purposes. She said she wasn't sure what is causing Stel's functionality problems, but that frequently doctors see brain tumor patients whose MRIs look pretty good but who aren't doing very well clinically. In Stel's case, her opinion was that there is a lot of "white matter change" throughout the brain on the recent MRI and this is the cause of Stel's current difficulties. Since I'd never heard of this problem and hadn't seen it mentioned as an issue in any previous MRI reports, I was rather taken aback and, of course, asked her what she meant. White matter change is abnormal tissue in the brain, probably the result of radiation therapy. It is probably permanent, she indicated. Needless to say, I was quite upset and confused, having never even contemplated this as an obstacle we'd run into.

As to the tumor itself, it is still stable and perhaps slightly smaller. My own comparison of the most recent scan to one taken in April before we left makes me think there may be some areas of change for the better that aren't noted in the radiologist's report (I won't get into technical details, but one does find oneself doing everybody's job when caring for a brain tumor patient). The only way to find out more specifically is to get another kind of MRI that can distinguish between live and dead tissue and I'm going to try to get that done in the next few weeks.

After my discussion with the surgeon, I spent some time looking back at previous MRIs and reports and found that in the April scan the same area that she referred to as "white matter changes" were noted as swelling by the previous radiologist. And the current radiologist noted that it is difficult to distinguish between the two. White matter changes simply weren't cited as an issue in any earlier reports. So I'm hoping we're dealing mostly with swelling here and I'm running around once again like a maniac getting copies of scans done so I can get them to other doctors here and elsewhere for their opinions. Maybe in three weeks' time or so I'll have some clarification, although it's also possible I'll just have a lot more confusion. We're supposed to go back to Mexico on July 31st for a follow-up vaccine shot and other treatment for a few days, but I'm unsure about that right now. Trying to travel with Stel when she's unable to function better is very difficult. And it's unclear whether the treatment is working for her. Her oncologist was impressed that the tumor is no larger and maybe a bit smaller given that it's been three months since Stel had any conventional treatment. It may be that the vaccine, etc. is working much more slowly for Stel than for others. I'm not yet ready to declare it a failure, but don't have any good evidence that it's an answer for Stel, either. So, as it has been throughout this awful fourteen-plus months, more horribly difficult decisions lie ahead.

How I wish I could send you a wonderful report that Stel is much better and improving daily. Unfortunately, that's not the case. She's still holding her own—eating well, looking pretty good for someone who's been through what she has (it was remarkable how many nurses and others at the hospital in Mexico said that Stel was beautiful, despite her steroid-swollen face and lack of hair)—but three weeks ago she stopped trying to talk at all. She hasn't talked a lot in past months except for isolated days, but I think this is the longest period she's gone without trying to utter a word. Needless to say, I don't know why and you can imagine how painful it is for me. This nightmarish journey continues on, with no clear path ahead. I'm still grateful for every day I have with Stella and the moments of happiness we have just being together. Kay

Tue Jul 04 2000 8:40 AM

Deborah, I'm sending you the message below separately so I could add this little note. I'm thinking fondly of Stel's birthday last year at your house. What a long year it's been. If you can come by at some point, give me a call. Love, Kay

Tue July 04 2000 8:57 AM

Dear George, This isn't the report I hoped I could send after our stay in Mexico, but I think the jury is still out on whether the treatment may be helpful. Now I'm not only worrying about the tumor but about "white matter changes" (see message below). I still hope for better days ahead. Kay

Wed Jul 05 2000 4:14 PM

Vanessa, Just got your message, so I'm forwarding the one I sent to everyone else yesterday. New information since I sent it is I'm getting Stel to Suburban Hospital within the hour because for the last 2-3 days she hasn't been taking her medications as she should and hasn't been drinking very much, so I asked the doctor to admit her to get this stuff through an IV. We need to get the steroid dose up high enough to see if it's going to help her become more alert—a sign we're dealing with swelling rather than white matter changes (see message below)—and I haven't been able to do that. Also, I want a neurologist to do some tests and see if s/he can alleviate some of the right-side spasticity and "spells" that Stel's been having and make some change in anti-seizure meds. The obstacles just keep coming and we just keep jumping. Needless to say, this is not the news I hoped to have after Mexico. But that's the way it goes—or the way Stel's life goes, anyway. Love, Kay

Wednesday, July 5, 2000

FAX to Dr. Howard Fine, NIH: I will bring to your office tomorrow MRI scans for Stelyani Sandris from 2/1/00, 3/12/00, 4/17/00 and 6/27/00 as well as copies of radiation and pathology reports you requested. These are my primary concerns about Stella at this point: Stella's surgeon does not think the 6/27 MRI shows a hydrocephalus problem severe enough to be causing her symptoms or to warrant putting in a shunt. She believes the symptoms are more likely caused by "extensive white matter changes" shown on the 6/27 scan. I would like to have your assessment of the significance of the hydrocephalus as well as whether we're dealing with white matter changes or edema or both.

Second, even though Stella's scans have been stable since the end of December, she has not been doing well clinically throughout that time. Since late January she really has not been able to do anything for herself and has no motivation. In the past three weeks, she has simply stopped trying to talk at all, although shortly before that she had some days when she was very responsive. Can you shed any light on why she's not doing better and give any suggestions on anything that might help her?

Third, within the past three months or so, she has become quite spastic on her right side and she has what I can only characterize as "right-side spells," where she draws her arm and leg up tight and stares off in space. She'll often make a sound as she tightens up her limbs. I've mentioned these occurrences to several doctors but haven't gotten any satisfaction in trying to find out what's going on and resolve the problem. I'd appreciate any help you can give us. Thanks, Kay Loveland

Sat Jul 08 2000 5:41 AM

Carole, I found out from the doctor that methylphenidate is Ritalin. The dosages the article recommends are significantly larger than what Stel was on. The neurologist is going to start her on 5 mg 2x a day and we'll see where we go from there. Kay

Sat July 08 2000 10:15 PM

Dear Dr. Friedman: We returned from Mexico a couple of weeks ago, and I'd like to send you some recent scans for review. Stel didn't respond to the vaccine as others have. CT scans and an MRI in San Diego indicated a hydrocephalus problem that doctors there thought was interfering with her response and making her sleepy, uncommunicative, and unable to hold her head up when she sat in the wheelchair. We had an MRI done when we got back and saw her surgeon. The surgeon thought Stel's difficulties are attributable to extensive white matter changes as shown on the latest scan. I'd like to send the scans to you for your review so you can tell me what you think.

The tumor itself appears to be about the same size as it was in April; it's really been stable since December. But Stel hasn't functioned well during this time. In the past three months, she has developed a lot of spasticity in her right limbs, whereas previously she had much more trouble on the left side (which she hasn't moved voluntarily in months), and has had what I refer to as right-side "spells" in which she draws up her right arm and leg quickly, holds them rigidly and stares off into space. About four weeks ago, she just stopped trying to speak at all. But she's still eating well and hasn't lost any weight. She's in the hospital here in Bethesda now. They've increased her Decadron to 36 mg a day to see if it helps.

The neurologist has checked for seizure activity and for restricted blood vessel flow and found neither. He started her on 10 mg of Ritalin today.

Please let me know if it's okay to send the scans to you for your input in the next few days. Thanks, Kay Loveland

Sun Jul 09 2000 6:12 AM

Dear Becky, I was at the memorial service yesterday. It was very moving and made me sorry I never met Dan. I wanted to stay to see you afterwards but had to leave quickly to run some errands and go back to Suburban Hospital, where Stel is now for some neurological tests and medications adjustments. It appears now that the reason she isn't functioning better despite a stable tumor for seven months may be brain damage from radiation. If the tumor doesn't get you, the treatment will with this horrible disease. I'm glad you have a lot of good friends, family, and support to help you get through this heart-wrenching time. Love, Kay

Sun Jul 09 2000 9:42 PM

Steve, The neurologist started Stel on Ritalin yesterday. She was more awake all day today than she's been for a while, but still mostly out in space somewhere and not making any effort to communicate. I expect she'll be in the hospital until at least next Wednesday. Kay

Mon Jul 10 2000 10:55 AM

Dear Ms. Loveland: I will send you a reprint of the article today. We have had many brain tumor patients with history of seizures on Ritalin and have not had any increase in seizures—there is an article cited in my work about lack of inducing seizures in patients with traumatic brain injury. We routinely up the dose to whatever it takes to get an effect; some patients are on 60 mg twice a day. Christina Meyers

Mon Jul 10 2000 6:39 PM

Dear Ms. Loveland: I have reviewed the MRI films. The degree of ventriculomegaly is impressive, and certainly out of proportion to any brain atrophy (the sulci are relatively normal). Although the periventricular edema could be due to radiation effect, it also could be linked to the hydrocephalus. The "bottom line" is that we have no effective medical/surgical treatment for radiation injury. It is possible that the corpus callosum glioma plus radiation have caused irreversible injury. However, I would definitely recommend that a palliative shunt be placed with the real possibility of regaining neurological function. Almost any neurosurgeon can place a shunt, and I would strongly recommend it. Good luck. Steven Brem, M.D., F.A.C.S.

Mon Jul 10 2000 11:23 PM

Dr. Brem: Thank you very much for your response. I'm surprised at the degree of disagreement between you and Stel's surgeon about the ventriculomegaly and will definitely seek out other opinions from surgeons in this area. Kay Loveland

Mon Jul 10 2000 11:28 PM

Carole, Stel was awake again today and toward evening watching a TV program she was interested in. The neurologist was pleased and is increasing her Ritalin dose to 10 mg twice a day tomorrow. He's also going to continue the B-12 shots beyond the three days that he had ordered as a result of my telling him about the AIDS dementia article. Keep fingers and toes crossed. Can you send the cite for that article about hyperbaric oxygen and radiation necrosis? Thanks, Kay

Tue Jul 11 2000 10:43 PM

Carole, Not as good a day today. Not sure what's happening. Hopefully, tomorrow will be better. Kay

Tue Jul 11 2000 11:18 PM

Dear Dr. Meyers: I called you today because I wanted to get more information about your experience with Ritalin and seizures in brain tumor patients that I could pass along to our neurologist. Three days ago he put my friend Stella on 5 mg of Ritalin twice a day. On Sunday and Monday, she was much more awake than she's been for some time and yesterday afternoon she seemed to be more focused and even watched part of a TV program, which she hasn't done in a while. (At the same time he put her on the Ritalin, he increased her Decadron to 36 mg a day.) Both the doctor and I were very pleased with what we saw yesterday and hoped today would be the same or better. He increased the Ritalin dose to 10 mg twice a day today.

Today, unfortunately, wasn't better. From early morning to late evening, Stella was mostly staring at the ceiling. (This started before she had her 10 mg dose in the morning.) I had a hard time getting her to focus on me when I talked to her. She also had some intermittent twitching of her leg that I couldn't stop and an occasional slight facial twitch. The neurologist immediately thought this indicated seizure activity caused by Ritalin. I told him that Stel had been staring at the ceiling for some time—well before she got Ritalin—although today was more consistent all day than I've seen it. He decided to leave the dose alone for today (she's already had 20 mg) and reassess tomorrow. I was upset that he immediately wanted to pull back on the Ritalin because from what we know now, it may be the only thing that offers promise to help her function a little better if, as it appears, we're dealing mostly with radiation necrosis problems instead of swelling. I believe in your article you indicated that you increased the Ritalin by 5 mg twice a day every two weeks. Do you consider that an optimum schedule to use? Could it be that he increased the dose too quickly (three days)? Have you encountered similar situations to the one I've described and, if so, did you feel it necessary to reduce the Ritalin dose? From your experience and to the extent you can tell from what I've told you, do you think what I've described is likely to be a result of taking Ritalin? If Stella has had this reaction already, does that mean she probably can't take a very high dose of it? You indicated in your message that you've treated many brain tumor patients with a history of seizures on Ritalin without any increase in seizures. Can you give me a ball park estimate of the numbers you've treated with this regimen? The neurologist says he doesn't pay much attention to studies because they only report the good results they've had and he said he'd seen studies that indicated there were problems with seizures on Ritalin. Are there such studies or was he just blowing hot air?

As is probably apparent, I'm very upset that he is so quick to abandon the Ritalin therapy (as was the previous neurologist) and really would appreciate any input you can give me. Perhaps he's right, but I'd like to have your insights on this if you feel comfortable in offering them. If you can call me tomorrow, that would be very helpful, since I'll be seeing him probably later in the afternoon. If this isn't convenient for you, an e-mail would be fine. Many thanks, Kay

Thu Jul 13 2000 11:04 PM

Carole, Can't tell you much more today than I could the other day. Stel hasn't been as alert and focused the last three days as she was Monday. Who knows why—not the neurologist, not I. Today she ate a large breakfast and lunch with gusto, and with her eyes closed. She had her eyes closed all day but was awake a good part of the time. Who knows why—not the neurologist, not I. She's still on a high dose of the steroid and he decided to go to 15 mg of Ritalin twice a day tomorrow. She's still in the hospital. I think we're going to put a tube in her stomach that is easier to manage than a port and that will enable me to give her just about anything in liquid form at home.

Her surgeon says she'll do a shunt or a temporary drain if I decide I want to do that, but she doesn't think it's likely to help much. I told her I'll decide about that after I get other opinions, especially from the neurosurgeon in L.A. whose opinion she would be interested in. Just got the scan off to him yesterday. Until later, Kay

Wed Jul 12 2000 10:01 PM

Dr. F: The scans from 4/17 and 6/27 should be there tomorrow morning. As I previously indicated, I'm interested to know what you and others there think about the significance of the ventriculomegaly and whether a shunt might be beneficial. Stel's surgeon and another doctor I've been in touch with disagree about this. Also, do you think the scans show extensive white matter change that is probably radiation damage and/or edema?

Stel is still in the hospital. The neurologist started her on 5 mg of Ritalin twice a day. She has been more awake for the past 3 days (but sleepier today) and on Monday she was quite alert. Yesterday she just stared at the ceiling all day. Today she did some staring and sleeping.

I'll appreciate hearing from you as soon as possible and having any recommendations you may have for where to go from here. I want to try to get an MRSpectroscopy soon. Thanks, Kay

Fri Jul 14 2000 8:31 AM

Re: Stel Sandris scans—shunt might be helpful but they should check the pressure in the spinal fluid before doing it. The tumor looks stable at the present time. Henry Friedman

Mon Jul 17 2000 5:33 AM

Dr. [David] Steenblock: I would like to know whether a brain tumor patient might benefit from your hyperbaric oxygen treatment. I'm attaching a summary of her medical history. As I note there, some doctors recently have said they believe she is suffering from delayed radiation injury. From the reading I have done, it appears to me that she has akinetic mutism. A neurologist did a doppler cranial exam on her last week and said that it showed the blood flow in her brain is okay. Consequently, he could not treat her with anti-coagulants as he had thought. He is treating her with Ritalin, which has been shown to be effective with brain tumor patients. So far she hasn't responded significantly to it. I'm wondering whether the fact that the cranial doppler showed normal blood flow would make her ineligible for hyperbaric oxygen treatment since one of its primary effects is in regenerating blood vessels. I would very much appreciate hearing from you as to whether you think you might be able to treat her with any likelihood of improvement. Thanks. Kay Loveland

Mon Jul 17 2000 6:01 AM

Kay, I got the articles, but both are old. Unless one of the doctors has specifically recommended using dopamine antagonists, they may want to see something newer than 1981. Dopamine antagonists are tricky, I understand. Love, Carole

Mon Jul 17 2000 6:14 AM

Carole, I'd like to see the old articles, as well as anything more recent on akinetic mutism, which appears to be what Stel is suffering from. The doctors seldom recommend anything; I've done most of the recommending. I have no idea what the neurologist's take on dopamine agonists is, but Ritalin is a mixed dopaminergic-nonadrenergic agonist. Thanks, Kay

Mon Jul 17 2000 12:55 PM

Dear Ms. Loveland: A doppler blood flow study only is good for detection of major blood vessel flow and says nothing about the microvascular flow. A sophisticated brain SPECT scan would be much better. I have treated radiation brain injuries before with good results. Sincerely, David Steenblock, DO

Tue Jul 18 2000 7:25 AM

Dr. Meyers, I'm sorry to keep pestering you, but I wondered whether you could tell me if you have patients on both Ritalin and anti-depressants like Paxil or Zoloft. It seems to me that perhaps they would offset each other. A neuro-oncologist I spoke with said he has treated many of his patients successfully with anti-depressants and he thinks one component of Stel's situation may be depression. I didn't get a chance to ask him whether he would give a patient Ritalin along with the anti-depressant. Would the Ritalin by itself have sort of an anti-depressant effect since it is a stimulant? Today Stella's dose is going to 25 mg twice a day. For the past couple of days she's been more awake and she's watched some TV quite intently. Much of the time, though, she's stared into space, and she's completely unresponsive to me and other people. Do you think we're seeing some response to Ritalin that will perhaps improve at higher doses, or if it kicks in will it do so all at once when we reach the right dosage? Any enlightenment you can give me on these questions will be deeply appreciated. Many thanks, Kay

Fri Jul 21 2000 7:00 AM

David, I'm sorry we couldn't talk when you called. My life continues at a frantic pace. It's a very difficult time because of lack of medical certainty over what is causing Stel's current problems and what, if anything, can be done to help her. Despite this, I continue to hope that things will get better soon. Thanks for calling, Kay

Wed Jul 26 2000 7:28 AM

Dear Natalie, I hope everything is going well for you there. Here, things continue to be frantic. Unfortunately, I don't have time to tell you much, but suffice it to say that Stella didn't respond to the treatment in Mexico as others have. This is probably because of other complications in her situation. I'm not sure at this point whether the vaccine has worked to keep the tumor stable and I'm still trying to sort things out so I can decide whether I should take her back to Mexico for follow-up treatment in a few weeks. In the meantime, she's been in the hospital here for three weeks—we just got out yesterday—for adjustment of medications and neurological tests. I've done my own research and think I have a pretty good idea of the problems she's suffering from and the possible remedies and I've been pushing the neurologist to give her meds that have helped others in her situation. Also, it's likely that I'm going to have to decide to have her surgeon put in a shunt.

I'm really discouraged and fed up with the doctors, none of whom are at all proactive and don't seem to know about the syndrome I believe she's got. They just look at her diagnosis and at the fact that she's not doing very well clinically and write her off—despite the fact that the tumor has been stable for seven months and she continues to eat well. So it's a fight every step of the way. Now the new neurologist who has been trying the drugs I've brought to his attention is balking at continuing to raise the dosages to levels that have helped others in studies I've shown him. It occurred to me that I need to see a psycho-pharmacologist. I remember your telling me about one you consulted. I would be extremely grateful if you could e-mail his name and phone number to me. Thanks so much. I can't tell you how much I miss seeing you (and Stella would, too, if she could speak) and how grateful I am for the lovely times you spent with Stella. Love, Kay

Sat Jul 29 2000 12:54 PM

Dear Dana, Thanks so much for your message. How wonderful it would be if Stel and I could be there enjoying the weather and the scenery and traveling with you and Karla. It breaks my heart to think it may never be possible for Stel to travel with me again. Unfortunately, I don't have any positive news. As usual, there were a few days in the hospital when I thought things were improving, but we came home Wednesday evening and since then Stel has been mostly sleeping and not responsive. It's so damned frustrating and heartbreaking. I'm completely fed up with the doctors here, none of whom really want to do anything. The neurologist I was working with on medications turned out to be a real jerk. I'd give anything to be in L.A. or San Francisco, or even Houston where M.D. Anderson is, now. This area is a wasteland for brain tumor treatment. I don't know what I'm going to do. Stel is now so weak from all her weeks in a hospital bed that it's practically impossible for me to handle her at home by myself. There are treatments and things I know of that I think could still help her, but I fear it's becoming physically impossible for me. If there were just one strong person who cared enough about Stel's life and could give some time to her, that's all I'd need. But that's impossible, too.

Despite her weakness and sleepiness, Stel is still eating pretty well and definitely distinguishes between food she likes and dislikes. That's my Stella, who loves good food. She's nowhere near dead, but the doctors are doing everything they can to write her off. I'll get a special MRI done on Wednesday, which will give me more information on how much of the tumor may be dead tissue now. I pray it won't show any new growth. I'm also going to talk to her surgeon this week about putting in a shunt since other doctors think it could help and the research I've done indicates to me that the fluid on the brain could be causing many of her problems. Sorry to go on with our troubles. Have a wonderful time there and know that Stel and I are with you in spirit. Love, Kay

Monday, July 31, 2000

MEMO to Drs. Neiman and Rajagopal: As you know, I have sought opinions from several other doctors regarding whether Stel might benefit from placement of a shunt. Those doctors have indicated that they think hydrocephalus may be a problem and that a shunt might be helpful. I want to set out a little more fully what they said. Dr. Steven Brem, chief of neurosurgery at Moffitt Cancer Center in Tampa, Florida stated: "The degree of ventriculomegaly is impressive, and certainly out of proportion to any brain atrophy.... I would definitely recommend that a palliative shunt be placed with the real possibility of regaining neurological function." Dr. Howard Fine, head of the Neuro-oncology Department at the National Cancer Institute said: "The only way to be sure about whether the enlarged ventricles indicate a hydrocephalus problem is to measure the pressure in the ventricles. It's not clear how much better, if at all, a shunt would make her if the pressure is basically normal." (He called hydrocephalus "the great masquerader" and went on to say that he believes Stel's myriad difficulties are a result of several things—possible radiation injury, hydrocephalus, bad location of tumor, and maybe seizure activity (apparently ruled out by EEGs) and depression. He didn't think that the white matter changes visible on Stel's MRI necessarily correlate with her condition. He's seen similar scans of patients who were functioning well.) Dr. Henry Friedman said a shunt might be helpful but that the CSF pressure should be tested first. In a phone conversation with Dr. Raj tonight, he indicated he thinks a shunt should be tried.

In the research I've done I've also found a number of articles regarding the syndrome of akinetic mutism, which appears to me to describe almost exactly what Stel has been suffering from for some time: "The patient sleeps more than normally, but is easily roused. In the fully developed state he makes no sound and lies inert...Despite his steady gaze, which seems to give promise of speech, the patient is quite mute, or he answers only in whispered monosyllables...There is total incontinence of urine and feces." There are several explanations for the cause of this syndrome, but the explanation that comes up most frequently is its association with obstructive hydrocephalus. One article states: "Hydrocephalus is a common denominator in many cases and not just an incidental finding. The importance of recognizing this syndrome, which is often remediable, cannot be overemphasized." I am wondering if whatever degree of hydrocephalus Stel may be suffering from could be a contributing factor to the condition of akinetic mutism she appears to be in. The studies indicate that patients with this syndrome have benefited from shunting and/or administration of anti-Parkinson's drugs. Ritalin has been used by doctors at M.D. Anderson to treat successfully hundreds of brain tumor patients, many afflicted with apathy syndrome. I'm enclosing some of the studies of akinetic mutism that I refer to.

While Stel was in the hospital during the last month, the neurologist started her on Ritalin and bromocriptine. Although there were a few days in the hospital when she seemed to be more alert and perhaps responsive to the medications, there has been no dramatic improvement as yet. However, I understand from the researcher at M.D. Anderson that they have gone as high as 60 mg of Ritalin twice a day to get a response, without any seizure problems. And the studies of bromocriptine indicate the patients who responded were on significantly higher doses than Stel is now on.

From all of this, I think I've reached the conclusion that trying a shunt is probably necessary. I'd appreciate talking to you this week about what course of action you would recommend. Are there tests you think it would be helpful to do? What are the risks? (I know we have touched on these in previous conversations, but I'd like to talk more concretely now.) I should note that Stel will be getting an MRSpectroscopy this week. Thanks. Kay

Tue Aug 08 2000 6:26 AM

Dear Dana, I appreciate your messages. Just a note to let you know that I think Stel will have surgery for placement of a shunt on Friday. I hate to have her go through it, but it appears to me to be the best chance she has of regaining some functioning. It will be more hell for me—watching and waiting to see what happens. Keep sending those prayers and positive thoughts our way. Love, Kay

Wed Aug 09 2000 7:22 AM

Dear Jean, I was interested to read about your father's fast walking problem. My partner Stel had the same problem last fall. Her oncologist thought swelling was causing it and increased her Decadron dose. It did seem to resolve after that, but then she began leaning far backward and could hardly walk in such a position. Somehow that ultimately resolved itself. Not long after that, she started falling and then couldn't walk at all. Now I'm in the midst of learning everything I can about "normal-pressure" hydrocephalus, which I believe Stel is afflicted with, and in the literature I've seen a couple of mentions of the leaning-forward phenomenon. Also, one of the things that happens with hydrocephalus is "gait disturbance" of various kinds and frequently it's the first sign of the problem. The other two signs are increasing mental difficulties and urinary incontinence—both of which Stel has had for some time, along with other problems. If I were you, I'd press this with your doctors. Stel's doctors never even mentioned hydrocephalus as a possibility. It should begin to show up on MRIs as an increase in the size of the ventricles, which it has for Stel, although until May "ventriculomegaly," as enlargement is called, was not even noted by the radiologists reading the MRIs, even though it was definitely there when I looked back at earlier scans. I've just decided this week to try a shunt for Stel, which will be done on this coming Friday. It's not a foregone conclusion that it will help her, but from what I've read it's had dramatic impact on many patients in her situation. I'm praying she'll finally have some luck. Good luck to you and your father. Kay

Wed Aug 09 2000 10:09 AM

Hi Kay! A dear friend of mine has a father afflicted with normal-pressure hydrocephalus. It is a very difficult condition to treat and he has not been doing well lately. He had a shunt installed several years ago and did very well, but a few months ago started having problems again (gait disturbances, incontinence, confusion). They did a shunt revision in June, but he is worse now than before the surgery. The doctors don't seem to know what to do about it. I found a website for her and I'm sending along the URL. It's a center at UCLA that specializes in normal-pressure hydrocephalus. I hope it gives you some info. Best of luck! Jody

Wed Aug 09 2000 5:45 PM

Dear Jody, Thank you so much. How I've wished Stel and I still lived in L.A., where we were for many years, instead of in the brain tumor wasteland of the Washington, D.C. area. I knew UCLA has a lot going on but had no idea they have a specific program for normal-pressure hydrocephalus. I'm trying to talk to the doctor in charge of it today to see whether I could get Stel out there (not an easy task without any help, but I'll do it) in a few days to have them look at her. I've already scheduled the shunt surgery for this Friday, but I'd feel a lot better to have her in the hands of people who are dealing with this all the time. Again, my thanks. Kay

Thu Aug 10 2000 6:53 AM

Dear Lynn, A very experienced neuro-oncologist at NIH [Dr. Howard Fine] told me he thought it unlikely that all of Stel's symptoms were caused by radiation injury to the frontal lobe (Stel's tumor started in right but moved somewhat across to left as well as through corpus callosum). He said this would be a diagnosis he would make only after ruling out other possibilities, one of which is, as he called it, "the great masquerader"—hydrocephalus. If Bob's MRIs show enlarged ventricles at all, then hydrocephalus could be implicated. I just learned yesterday about a program at UCLA that focuses on adult hydrocephalus and, in particular, normal-pressure hydrocephalus. I'm looking into it. I'll put the URL below. Good luck. Kay

Thu Aug 10 2000 10:58 AM

Jody, I just postponed Stel's surgery and the surgeon, despite protestations to the contrary, seemed rather put out. I was surprised. I thought she was more mature about these things. I told her I had just learned about the UCLA program and had to check it out before I could think of proceeding here. You'd think that would be understandable in these terrible circumstances we have to deal with, but ego still seems to rear its head. I hope desperately I can talk to the doctor at UCLA today and find out how soon I could get Stel into their program. Kay

Thu Aug 10 2000 11:16 AM

Dear List: I sent Dr. Friedman an e-mail asking about getting an MR Spec when we go back to Duke at the end of the month. His answer was and I quote, "MRI Spec is of marginal benefit…unless the MRI is worrisome then I would probably order a PET scan instead." I thought a Spec showed the chemical makeup of the tumor. After going back and reading about both, I'm not sure. Which does what? I'm totally confused now. Anyone out there had a PET scan done? Debra

Fri Aug 11 2000 6:29 AM

Debra, My partner Stel just had a PET scan yesterday. We should get results today, so we'll see. We got this scan after she had an MR Spec last week which the radiologist said he wasn't able to read. He couldn't explain why they weren't able to get readable Spec pictures but suggested that a PET scan would be better anyway. (The PET takes several hours, during which time the patient has to lie perfectly still. The MR Spec is an MRI with a little additional time added to do the Spec part.) I know I've seen a lot of differing opinions among doctors and others as to which type of scan is most useful for differentiating necrosis from live tumor, with some favoring MR Spec and some PET. I'm interested to know that Dr. Friedman favors PET. Hoping for promising results. Kay

Fri Aug 11 2000 8:20 PM

Dear Jody, Unfortunately, the doctor hasn't called me back as of 5 p.m. L.A. time today. I called three times yesterday and twice today to no avail. The woman who answered the phone this afternoon assured me he had my messages. Part of the problem is that the woman who handles scheduling isn't there. She'll be back Monday and I hope can answer some of my questions and get the doctor to call me about the others. But until then I've got to stew about it over the weekend. What makes me feel worst is delaying getting anything done for more weeks because this has been hanging fire for a couple of months now, and I just can't bear to see Stel just lying in the bed sleeping or awake but mute and unable to do anything. I want so much to help her regain some functioning. It just breaks my heart that the tumor has been stopped in its tracks for seven months but Stel hasn't had any benefit from it. She's just lost one function after another until now she's got no life—and neither do I.

I can't be sure that it's normal-pressure hydrocephalus that is causing most of her problems, but from everything I've read on the subject, it sure seems to fit. Her surgeon here is skeptical and has been discouraging. I long to be where there's a team of doctors working on the problem and not one lone surgeon and one lone neurologist who won't read the research I give them and aren't up on the latest information or tests. I'm impressed, too, with UCLA's testing program and feel I owe it to Stel to look into it more fully. So I hate sitting here twiddling my thumbs letting time pass because I'm not able to talk to anyone there. It's going to be a very difficult weekend. I'm also going to be fretting over the results of a PET scan Stel had yesterday. The report was supposed to be ready this afternoon, but I've heard nothing from the doctor, so now I'm stuck on that until Monday, too. Sorry. I'm feeling pretty low tonight. All I can tell you is that a neutron bomb has been dropped on Stel's and my life of 31 years together. The bodies are left, but the life is gone—at least at the present. In my better moments I still hope to regain some of it. Tonight I'd just as soon jump out the window if I could.

We live near the D.C. line in Bethesda, Maryland. Stel never liked it here and I feel so bad that this terrible thing has happened to her here. We're pretty stranded because the friends who could be of most help are on the West Coast. Also, this is not the place to be with a brain tumor. Doctors with expertise are hard to come by. Johns Hopkins is pretty close, but still a schlep, and we went there a couple of times early in the game and found it depressing and conservative. As I said before, what I'd give to be living in L.A. now. Thanks so much for your messages. They mean a lot. Kay

Fri Aug 11 2000 8:29 PM

Dana, I wanted to let you know that I postponed the surgery while I check into a program at UCLA I just found out about that specializes in the problem Stel has. I felt I had to talk to the doctor there before proceeding here. I just don't feel comfortable with the way it has been approached by her surgeon; she keeps emphasizing the negatives, in particular the difficulty of setting the pressure correctly and the danger of subdural hematomas. I'm sure she'd do a good job on the surgery but I'm more concerned about the follow-up and feeling like the burden is all on me. Unfortunately, I haven't been able to talk to the doctor in L.A. and have to go through the weekend now. These are very hard times and I'm feeling very alone tonight, so I was glad to hear from you. Will this deluge of ill fortune never let up? Kay

Sat Aug 12 2000 7:37 AM

Dear Mary, I'm so sorry to hear about your sister. As to how Stel's doing, it's a long, involved story—the bottom line of which is I don't know at this point. For several weeks, I ran around getting doctors' opinions on whether Stel is afflicted with hydrocephalus and whether a shunt might help. Most of them said they thought so. Her surgeon had an opposite opinion but, after hearing the other doctors' opinions, said she would do it if I wanted her to even though she's still skeptical it will work. I've done a lot of research in the last several weeks on "normal-pressure hydrocephalus," which seems to be the most likely affliction and found that's very difficult to diagnose and doesn't always respond to shunts, but when it does, the recovery of function is dramatic. Also, I've found some research on the successful use of Ritalin and anti-Parkinson's drugs to treat some of Stel's many problems. But getting the doctors here to pay attention to this stuff is practically impossible. I had decided to go ahead with the shunt surgery yesterday and then on Wednesday night found out about a UCLA program that specializes in normal-pressure hydrocephalus. I felt I owed it to Stel to check into this so I postponed the surgery and have been trying to reach the doctor at UCLA for a couple of days. I don't know what I'll do about getting her to L.A. if it looks like the best thing to do. She's weaker now than she was when we went to Mexico because she's had no physical therapy in three months and she has the problem of not being able to keep her head up. But I"ll deal with the logistics if I think it is the best thing for her. What concerns me is follow-up after the surgery when there could be complications. I just don't feel I have any support from the doctors here.

The heartbreaking thing, among many, is even though the tumor has been stable for months, Stel has had a progressive loss of function to the point now where she doesn't even try to talk. She's still eating well and enjoying good food, but that's her only pleasure. It's just horrible.

I'm still not sure whether the vaccine from Mexico has worked. The tumor didn't appear to be much smaller on the recent MRIs. But we had a PET scan done this week and I'm awaiting the results of that—praying that it will show a lot of dead tissue. I'm hoping beyond hope for some good news next week. If there is a lot of dead tumor, I'd be inclined to think that the vaccine had something to do with that since Stel hasn't had any conventional treatment since the end of March. And if the vaccine is working, we need to go back for a follow-up shot soon, which is another big logistical question.

That's the frantic story from here for the moment. We just keep on keeping on, but it's very difficult. I feel like every obstacle that could be thrown in my path has been, and unfortunately I've got no one to help me. Stel's family is completely hopeless. My family is only marginally better. The friends who could be most helpful are on the West Coast. I'll let you know if we head to L.A. All the best, Kay

Sat Aug 12 2000 7:42 AM

Lynn, Given my experience with Stella—her tumor has been stable for seven months but she's progressively lost function, starting back last fall with the fast walking—and the research I've recently done on what may be afflicting her, I'd say to keep pressing your doctors to come up with better answers. I think they too often just say, well this is a brain tumor and this is what happens when, in fact, there are other problems causing the symptoms—like hydrocephalus, which one doctor I talked to recently called "the great masquerader." Good luck, Kay

Sun Aug 13 2000 10:49 AM

Dear Kay, Got your e-mail about postponing the surgery. I do think it was wise to do so if you had reservations about it. Stel is getting so weak that I know you don't want to do anything to further that. I again hope you get good news or at least some encouragement from the UCLA doctor to proceed as you have planned. That would at least give you more peace of mind. I'm sure not surprised that you have had a 'down' night. You are not only physically exhausted but mentally you must be on overload. What you are doing is usually not humanly possible. You are the sole caregiver and the sole investigator for brain tumors. Kay, please, please try to get some rest. Stel would be the first to tell you that if she could. The other thing she would tell you would be that she loves you and that you couldn't have done anything more to help her. You have exhausted all possibilities and I know that you won't let up for even a second. But I am concerned for my sister, too. Love you, Dana

Sun Aug 13 2000 5:41 PM

Dear Vanessa, Thank you for your offer of housing and help. Fortunately, I think there are a few people in L.A. I can call upon for such things and it's comforting to know you are among them. The more I hear from people on the BT List about treatment at UCLA, the more I think it's the place Stel might get the attention she needs. She's sure not getting it here. I think I can still manage to get her there if necessary, but it will require a lot of logistical maneuvering.

No, to my deep heartache, Stel isn't communicative at all. June 2nd was the last day she tried to talk much and she was laughing at jokes in a Steve Martin movie she had to understand in order to respond, and laughing with nurses at the hospital in Mexico. Shortly thereafter, all words, smiles and laughs ceased. After having done frantic research, I discovered she's probably afflicted with a condition called "akinetic mutism," which is often associated with hydrocephalus. I won't go into all the ins and outs that led me to the UCLA hydrocephalus program, but because of the difficulties of diagnosing and treating the condition, I'm very interested in talking to the doctors there to see whether the program might be helpful to Stel.

The heartbreaking thing is that Stel might have had some decent life these last months if the doctors had helped me figure out what was wrong. I kept asking and looking for the right doctors here but never found them. Needless to say, if I could have foreseen the future, we never would have left L.A. It's just a dreadful situation and I've been going through hell for weeks. Do I have some help? A home health aide for a couple of hours three times a week and a visiting nurse once or twice a week. Volunteers for 2-3 hours just about every day. But I'm going to have to hire people soon to free up more hours for me. Once I get the next step figured out, I'll think about that. Again, my thanks. Kay

Sun Aug 13 2000 5:49 PM

Dear Kay, What an anxiety-provoking situation. It sounds like the right decision to postpone the surgery until you see what UCLA can offer. Once again, all of your research and efforts have paid off. It sounds as if you're moving heaven and earth to get an answer. Let me know what happens with the scan. Is Stel in the hospital at the moment? Deborah

Mon Aug 14 2000 11:45 PM

Steve, Can't go into details now, but I had to take Stel to the emergency room today because she was breathing very hard. We were in the ER most of the day—mostly waiting. They did a CT scan and said the hydrocephalus appears to have increased a bit. This might be causing pressure on the brain stem and making her have a harder time with respiration. The oncologist thinks the breathing may be related to pneumonia or an infection and is doing tests. I talked to UCLA and found out there's no way Stel could get treated there for a couple of months. Of course, I couldn't take Stel anyway when she has breathing problems and is on oxygen. They said they'd do a mail consultation but I think circumstances have changed now with the breathing and the increased hydrocephalus and I don't want to wait around another couple of weeks, so I think the surgery will go ahead pretty soon. However, the surgeon is acting weird. I thought she was going to come by to talk to me tonight and she didn't. The oncologist did and said she had talked to the surgeon who indicated she didn't think she was involved because I was taking Stella to UCLA (even though I had told her assistant who looked at the CT scan today that I wanted to see her and proceed with the surgery). Ah, these doctors and their egos. The patient gets lost in the shuffle. So it goes in the surreal brain tumor world. Gotta get to bed. I'll phone you tomorrow. Kay

Wed, Aug 16 2000 7:27 AM

Dear Deborah, Stel is back in the hospital as of Monday. Her breathing became a bit labored and she had a little temperature so the doctor admitted her. They did a CT scan which showed that the hydrocephalus was perhaps increased a little. They put her on oxygen to help her breathing. Given these circumstances, I decided to go ahead with the shunt surgery as soon as possible. It would have been Thursday or Friday but now they've found a possible blood infection they've got to treat with antibiotics for 7-10 days first. I did check with the UCLA program and found out that, even if I could get her there, it would be two months before they could take her as an in-patient. I just wish I'd known about the program six weeks ago when I was running around getting opinions. Her surgeon remains the most pessimistic of all the doctors about whether a shunt will help and continues to believe we're dealing with radiation damage. What I'd give to have Stel treated at a center like UCLA but there's no way to get her there now. Hopefully, we'll have a chance later. Kay

Wed Aug 16 2000 9:42 PM

Dr. Friedman, Stel had a PET scan done last week and I'm sending a copy down to you tomorrow. I'd appreciate a reading by your people at Duke. Report from here is it's "consistent with viable tumor in midline area and on either side of large defect in cortical gray matter." However, I'm wondering if more information can be gleaned from the scan—how much supposed tumor versus necrosis in tumor area? And, given her surgeon's belief that the extensive white matter changes shown on her last MRI reflect permanent radiation necrosis/damage, I'm wondering whether the PET scan can tell us anything about necrosis in other areas of the brain. I'd appreciate any further light that might be shed on these questions. Thanks, Kay

Fri Aug 18 2000 4:23 PM

Dear Kay, It makes us sick to think about what you are having to endure right now. War zone in the soul! Where are you now drawing your strength from? When does a human run dry? I am so impressed by what you are giving, Kay. 100 percent sacrificial love. And I think that you are using extremely good judgment about Stel's treatment. Just the fact that you research so much and seek so many opinions, that is far beyond what most people do. Stel is in the best hands with you. One of the last things she wrote to me is how grateful she is that you are there for her. Mom turned to me today and said, "I wish Kay were here right now, she would love this," and I knew she was right—BUT you are fulfilling a MUCH higher duty. I am praying for you. Much LOVE, Karla

Fri Aug 18 2000 10:23 PM

Dear Karla, Thank you for your message. It is a terrifying and exhausting journey that Stel and I are on, but my deep love for her renews my strength and resolve day by day. Among the most disheartening and fatiguing aspects of it is having to fight not only the tumor and all its manifestations, but the pessimism of the doctors here. They do a great disservice to people in Stel's situation by always painting the blackest picture they can and I'm sure they kill people with their pessimism. I'm determined they won't do that to Stel.

Today Stel was very alert, her beautiful brown eyes were sparkling and following me and others as we talked. At one point, when I was having a conversation with someone about things I now believe were tumor-related that happened before we knew she had it, she opened her eyes and looked directly at me and clearly was interested in what I was saying. She's there and we've just got to help her get back. She's breathing much better and the blood infection seems to be going away. But the antibiotic regimen runs fourteen days and I don't know whether she'll be able to have the shunt surgery before that has fully run its course. If not, it wouldn't be until week after next. Whenever it's going to be, I'm now having to deal with the quandary of whether to change neurosurgeons again. The one we've had acted like such a jerk about my postponing the surgery last week—which probably was for the best since the blood infection probably started about that time. She has it in her mind now that I'll never be satisfied and if the shunt doesn't work, as she has never thought it would, then I'll insist on lowering the pressure to try to get it to work, which could result in blood clots on the brain.

We had a long talk about all this and worked through her misperceptions, I think, but I'm concerned that her attitude toward me might make working with her difficult after the surgery is done. Also I just saw her before I left the hospital to come home for a while and once again she's so goddamned negative that I just want to scream. She had suggested that maybe I should talk to another neurosurgeon and I decided that might be a good idea, so I met with one that she asked to come around. He seemed easier to talk to about the research I've done, and more interested in it, but I think his attitude about the effectiveness of a shunt is also pretty negative. I want to talk to him on Monday more about this. I'm concerned that our current surgeon's strong bias that Stel is suffering from irreversible radiation damage and is in an inexorable decline will cause her not to try as hard as she could after the shunt is put in to make it effective if, in fact, it isn't effective at first. And I want to know if he shares her views, how strong is his bias in that direction.

This whole week has been filled with unnecessary frustrations and difficulties and this nonsense with the surgeon topped the list. I wish so much that Stella and I could be there to share the good times with all of you. I'm still hoping that day will come. Love, Kay

Sat Aug 19 2000 1:44 PM

Dear Deborah, The infection seems to be on its way out, but now I'm told by the surgeon that the antibiotic is a fourteen-day cycle and she wouldn't recommend doing the surgery until it's run its course. The oncologist thinks it would be okay after ten days as long as they keep giving Stel the antibiotic for fourteen. On top of this, because of the problem I had with Stel's surgeon about postponing the surgery, I'm now faced with deciding whether I want her or a new surgeon to do the operation. She suggested I might want to talk to another surgeon. I didn't think so at first because I know she would do the best job that could be done on the surgery itself, but then I began to think that if another surgeon had a less pessimistic view, that would be good. I met with a surgeon she asked to come by, but I've got to talk to him more before I make a decision.

I'm so damned sick of the negativity of the doctors here (except for the oncologist; her partners are negative, but she's always more upbeat). They look at Stel for a couple of minutes, look at her scans a couple of seconds and they're ready to pronounce her all but dead. If I hadn't done all the reading I've done about akinetic mutism and normal-pressure hydrocephalus, I wouldn't have a clue that maybe their negativism is misplaced. I've lived this 24 hours a day for months and having read the case histories, I can only say that what Stel has experienced tracks very closely with what the patients afflicted with these syndromes went through. Couple that with MRIs and CT scans that have several indicia of hydrocephalus, and it seems to me more likely than not that that's what is causing many of Stel's difficulties. If she isn't afflicted with it, she's doing a damned good imitation of it. I've just got to keep these doctors from killing Stel with their pessimism.

Meanwhile, the almost-dead one was very alert yesterday and this morning. Her eyes were wide open and bright and sparkly and she was following me and others with her eyes and paying attention when I talked to her, even watched a little TV. And, as usual, she ate a good breakfast. She's there and we've got to release her from the trap she's in.

The special scan I had done hasn't yet enlightened me much. I sent it to Duke with questions and hope maybe I'll get more answers, but I'm not holding my breath. [I never did get the answers I sought.] It appears from the MRI taken early this month that the tumor area continues to be essentially the same size. But I'm worrying constantly about what to do about treatment for that. The neuro-oncologist at Duke said since the tumor is stable we should wait until the shunt is put in before deciding on more chemo since the chemo damages tissue, too. If Stel improves with the shunt, which according to the literature could be within a matter of days or a couple of weeks (but her surgeon said it could take many weeks), then we'd know she's not suffering from irreversible brain damage that chemo would add to. Of course, there's still the whole question of whether to try to follow up with the vaccine if possible because I still have no clear indication as to whether it has or hasn't had an effect.

Sorry to go on, but you caught me at a moment when I was stewing about these damned doctors and needed to let off steam to someone. Love, Kay

Sat Aug 19 2000 9:46 PM

Emily, I just wanted to let you know that I have completed half of the manual as of this week, except for some minor changes I still need to make, and will turn that over to David in early September unless I receive other instructions. I'm continuing to make steady progress and fully expect to complete the work in late October or early November. Kay

Mon Aug 21 2000 5:53 AM

Carole, Stel has done remarkably well for the past three days, especially yesterday. Wide awake much of the day, eyes alert and following people, even moving her head a little, which I haven't seen in quite a while. I would have sworn she was going to say something a couple of times. I'm hoping for a fourth day. Kay

NOTE: Even though I had already decided to go ahead with the shunt after Stel was taken to the ER on August 14th, I still wanted to have the specialists in hydrocephalus at UCLA give me their opinion and therefore wrote the following letter:

Monday, August 21, 2000

LETTER to Dr. Marvin Bergsneider, Director, UCLA Adult Hydrocephalus Center: I am enclosing MRI scans for Stelyani Sandris from March, April, and August 2000, as well as reports on those scans. I'm also attaching a chronology over the the past several months that sets out her progressive loss of function. From the case histories I have read regarding people afflicted with normal pressure hydrocephalus, it seems to me that Stel's experience tracks many of them quite closely. I would appreciate receiving an opinion from you as to the likelihood that Stel is suffering from normal pressure hydrocephalus. Because of extensive white matter changes seen on her MRI scans, her surgeon is inclined to believe that the cause of her lack of functioning is radiation injury. I look forward to your response. Sincerely, Kay Loveland

Wed Aug 23 2000 10:20 PM

Dr. Friedman: Did you get the PET scan I sent down last week? Any reading? Thanks, Kay

Thu Aug 24 2000 8:08 AM

[To Kay Loveland]: Looks like active tumor but need an MRI to correlate it with. Henry [Friedman]

Thu Aug 24 2000 11:31 AM

Gail, What do you mean when you say you think "neurosurgeons see hydrocephalus in a more pronounced state"? I ask because for two months I've been hassling with my partner's neurosurgeon about whether hydrocephalus is causing many functional problems that she has. Her NS has been quite negative about it, but another neurosurgeon and a neuro-oncologist who has looked at a lot of these scans are more positive. Stel is now scheduled to have shunt surgery on Monday after I've done a lot of research and gone back and forth on it for quite a while. As a NS said to me yesterday, "We're not really talking science here; we're talking a judgment call." I'm interested in knowing more about your experience. Thanks, Kay

Sun Aug 27 2000 9:26 PM

Cathy, Just wanted to let you know that Stel will have surgery for placement of a shunt early tomorrow morning. If it works, it should help her a great deal. She has been doing well this last week—much more awake and alert, those beautiful brown eyes radiating the personality trapped inside. She's even watched a couple of movies all the way through, which she hasn't done in quite a while, and today she made a couple of small sounds when I was talking to her that I know were efforts to communicate. It's so touching and heartrending.

I don't know how long they'll let her stay in the hospital after the surgery. The usual is a couple of days. I don't feel very comfortable bringing her home that quickly without a lot more help, so she may go to another facility for recuperation and, hopefully, some rehab. Love, Kay

Mon Aug 28 2000 2:09 PM

Dear Peter, Stel came through the surgery well. Now it's a matter of watching, waiting, and hoping to see signs of improvement. Could take days or weeks (her surgeon keeps talking about weeks) and may require adjustment of pressure down the road. I'm hoping we'll see something positive in a few days, which has happened with patients I've read about. But I fear to get my hopes up and have them dashed to the ground again. We're still in the same hospital room probably through tomorrow. Then I'm not sure whether we'll be home or at a nursing home for a week or so of recuperation. I'd like to have a few more days in a facility before I bring her home, but the decision lies in the insurance company's hands. Kay

Tue Aug 29 2000 5:03 PM

Mary, Thanks so much for your message. Stel came through the surgery fine and hasn't had any problems afterward. Now it's more watching and waiting for me and I'm terrified nothing will happen. This is truly living hell. But thank god she's not in any pain and the tumor up to the latest MRI three weeks ago remains stable. And I do my best to put my fears to the back of my mind and just keep hugging and kissing her and telling her I love her, and the moments when she looks back deeply into my eyes are worth more than any fortune I could ever have. I'm hoping for good luck finally to shine on my Stella. I appreciate deeply your thoughtfulness. Kay

Tue Aug 29 2000 5:58 PM

Tracy, I've had the same experience you've had with your dad—doctors saying my partner Stel is ready for hospice. I know she's not; and I know the tumor has not been growing for several months. Her problems aren't problems of dying; they're problems that need to be dealt with so she can live better. You have to fight the doctors' nihilism about this disease. It's too easy in this brain tumor world to give up on people, especially where a GBM is involved. At the same time we're struggling against the tumor and all the myriad ramifications of it, we have to struggle against the profound pessimism of the doctors. I'm very wary of deciding that someone whose brain is playing tricks on them is ready to die. There are a variety of reasons for why someone with a BT might have mental deterioration and they don't all lead to death. And I know Stel and know she wants me to fight for her life, which I will do with every ounce of strength I have. If you feel similarly, you shouldn't let doctors talk you into making a decision you don't think is right. Keep on keeping on. Kay

Wed Aug 30 2000 5:12 AM

Dear Jody, Glad to hear your dad is a little better. I think in this horrible situation we all face it's too easy to decide the end is near. As I've learned, there can be more than one reason why a person may appear to be on a downhill slide. But then they do something that surprises us. I tend to agree with your mother: If the color looks good—and especially if the person still wants to eat—there's hope. So hang in there. You never know what can happen in this surreal world we inhabit.

Stel's doing fine after the surgery. No signs yet of any improvement and I'm terrified I'll be waiting and hoping and nothing will happen. But I do my best to put those fears out of my mind. I hug and kiss her and tell her I adore her, and I keep hoping that good fortune finally will come Stella's way. Kay

Thu Aug 31 2000 5:37 AM

Deborah, Stel came through the surgery fine. She's had no post-operative problems. The doctor said she was able to position the shunt perfectly. Now the even harder part, for me, comes—waiting and hoping. Dr. Neiman talks about waiting weeks to see if Stel responds (even so, she came in the first morning after and asked if there were any changes); the research I've read speaks of days up to two weeks to see positive changes. The first couple of post-op days were a little worse than the days before the surgery when Stel often was tracking with her eyes and paying attention to things and making some small sounds that seemed to be efforts to communicate. Yesterday she just mainly stared into space. So god knows if and when things will change for the better, and I don't know how I'm going to bear more of this, but I have no choice. Of course, after we've waited some weeks we may have to adjust the pressure in the shunt and then watch and wait some more. Sheer hell.

I was able to get the insurance company to approve a five-day stay in a nursing home for more recuperation before I bring Stel home, so we'll go to a place very close to where we used to live today through Monday. Thanks for staying in touch. Kay

Thu Aug 31 2000 6:02 AM

David, I'm planning to turn over to you next week the first half of the manual, which I've completed. I'll probably ask someone to bring the disk in for me. If you have any questions or concerns, let me know by e-mail or phone. Kay

NOTE: I received the following letter from Dr. Bergsneider at the UCLA Hydrocephalus Center in early September, several days after Stel's shunt surgery. I wished that I had found out about the Center much earlier and had received Dr. Bergsneider's opinion before I felt pressed to make a decision after Stel was taken to the ER in mid-August. If I had, I think I would have decided against a shunt.

Thursday, August 31, 2000

LETTER from Dr. Marvin Bergsneider, Director of the UCLA Adult Hydrocephalus Center: Dear Ms. Loveland, The question that you pose to me, does Stelyani Sandris have normal pressure hydrocephalus, requires a complex answer. Given the limited data available to me, it is not possible to say that hydrocephalus is definitely not responsible for some of her symptoms and signs. It is important to note that the signs and symptoms of NPH are not specific. In your letter you state that her findings "track" the experience of others. Although this may be true to some degree, NPH is a syndrome that must be considered in context. Nine out of ten patients with gait instability, bladder dysfunction, and/or memory problems do not have NPH. Therefore the fact that someone has suggestive findings does not make the diagnosis.

Although the MRI scans do show some degree of ventricular enlargement, the other changes to the brain are rather profound. There is extensive white matter changes in the cerebrum bilaterally that is not consistent with so-called transependymal edema (due to hydrocephalus). Also, tumor is clearly bihemispheric affecting the mesiofrontal lobes. This is the specific area of the brain that is affected by hydrocephalus. Therefore, I feel that it is much more likely that the combination of the tumor and radiation-induced white matter destruction is responsible for her symptoms. Having said that, you may wonder if hydrocephalus is adding insult to injury. It may be, but my experience treating possible hydrocephalus in cases similar to your friend has been very disappointing. Little if any improvement was seen, and the complication rate was high. For some patients, they were left worse off than prior to the shunt. This is not a case of "what harm can it do?" I feel for the suffering you and your friend are going through and apologize if my opinion is not what you wanted to hear. I wish you the best. Sincerely, Marvin Bergsneider, M.D.

Fri Sep 01 2000 5:02 AM

Friends, Stel is now in a nursing home for further recuperation for five days. The first couple of days after the surgery, which went fine, haven't been encouraging. I had hoped at least for status quo ante because Stel was pretty alert for the week or so before the surgery. But yesterday and the day before, she just stared into space. This may mean nothing and at any moment she could snap back, as I've seen her do before, but it's the longest period of time that she's done this. Also, they tried to take her off the oxygen before we left the hospital but had to put her back on it (at a low level) because her saturation level fell off. Who knows what this all means? I don't; the doctors don't. I can only tell you it's extremely painful. So far as I know now, we'll be at the nursing home until Tuesday. I wish I had better news to send you. Love, Kay

Fri Sep 01 2000 9:03 PM

Emily, I'll be glad to have the disk delivered to John. However, as I indicated, I will need to have it returned to me as soon as possible so I can continue making changes to the text of the remainder of the manual. I'll arrange for someone to bring the disk into the office next week. Kay

Fri Sep 01 2000 9:10 PM

Friends, Today was slightly more encouraging than the couple of days before. Stel slept for a lot of the day but when she was awake didn't stare into space until late this evening just before I left. I wish I could pray for strength to get me through these days, but since I can't, I just have to keep on keeping on. Kay

Fri Sep 01 2000 10:29 PM

Dear Kay, After being on the List for two years, I have seen levels of commitment between family/partners. You are at the top of my list as one of the most devoted. (I'm sure you're saying, "Well, of course, I love Stel!") Janet

Sat Sep 02 2000 5:00 AM

Dear Janet, Thank you for the kind words. Quite a few people have said similar things to me throughout this terrifying odyssey Stel and I have been on. So far as

I am concerned, I can't imagine doing any less and only wish I could do more. Stel deserves it, and she would do the same for me. Best wishes, Kay

Tue Sep 05 2000 5:32 AM

Dr. Friedman: I thought my previous e-mail may have gotten lost in the shuffle. Did you get the MRI I sent week before last and have a chance to look at it in conjunction with the PET scan? Stel had a shunt placed a week ago. So far no signs of improvement. She'll have another MRI next Monday, which I'll send down as soon as possible. I then want to see about moving ahead with some further drug treatment. Thanks, Kay

Tue Sep 05 2000 8:17 AM

[To Kay Loveland]: We never got it but will check again today. Henry [Friedman]

Thu Sep 07 2000 4:23 AM

Dr. F: Please let me know if you haven't found it so I can have Fed Ex trace it. Thanks, Kay

Thu Sep 07 2000 8:22 AM

[To Kay Loveland]: Got the stuff located—apparently Duke sent the prior MRI back—looks similar by memory but not as good as doing a side by side. Henry [Friedman]

Thu Sep 07 2000 7:41 PM

Dr. F: Sorry, I don't quite understand your message. I take it you found the current MRI but not the previous one? (Duke didn't send it back to me.) What about comparison to PET scan? Sorry to take up your time with this. Thanks, Kay

Thu Sep 07 2000 7:46 PM

Carole, We came home yesterday. No news. Stel was pretty alert yesterday afternoon; even ate a little dinner. Today she's been very sleepy, although she ate a very good breakfast. The same old roller coaster ride. I'm feeling very lonely and bleak at the moment. Thanks for the thoughts. Kay

Fri Sep 08 2000 9:31 AM

[To Kay Loveland]: There is activity which could be tumor or rt damage. No way to tell. Henry [Friedman]

Sat Sep 09 2000 10:03 AM

Dr. F: Sorry. One more question: Are you saying that the activity that showed up on the PET scan could be radiation damage instead of tumor, even though the doctor who read it at Georgetown said it was consistent with active tumor? I know the MRI doesn't differentiate but I thought the PET was supposed to give us a better idea, even though it's far from 100% accurate. Kay

Sat Sep 09 2000 5:57 PM

[From Dr. Friedman]: PETs cannot differentiate RT damage from tumor unless the PET is cold. Hypermetabolism can be seen with either—however, tumor is more likely. Henry

Wed Sep 13 2000 6:34 AM

Nancy, Thanks for the visit. It helped a lot. Drop by whenever you can. Stel's MRI on Monday showed the tumor is still stable. The doctor took her stitches out and lowered the pressure another couple of notches. More watching, waiting, and hoping. Kay

Thu Sep 14 2000 5:21 AM

Carole, In addition to articles on radiation necrosis, please check for anything on radiation damage or injury, which is different from necrosis. I'd like to see the comments on the warfarin-heparin article. Keep a watch, too, for more stuff on Ritalin and anti-Parkinson's or dopamine agonists. In addition to bromocriptine, I've seen mention of Cogentin, Prolopa, amantadine hydrochloride. Another drug mentioned—not sure it's a dopamine agonist—is physostigmine. Also ephedrine. Christina Meyers said they're also trying modafinil (Provigil) and have used Aricept (Alzheimer's drug). There was mention on the BT List of someone trying pentoxyfilline (Trental) for radiation necrosis. Might also check on antidepressants or anti-psychotics used for apathy. I'd like to look at stuff they're using for stroke patients as well. Thanks, Kay

Thu Sep 14 2000 9:53 PM
RE: HIT BY A NEUTRON BOMB

Dear Friends [on BT List], It's been a long time since I've posted an update on my partner Stel's situation. That's partly because as the sole caregiver I haven't found the time in the midst of a whirlwind of hospitalizations, consultations, research, and decisions, partly because it's been so unclear to me what is going on that I didn't know what to say, and partly because I feel like our lives have been hit by a neutron bomb during the past several months—the bodies are still here but the life we had is destroyed—and I'm so heartbroken that I don't know if I can put our experience into words. If you want to know more about normal-pressure hydrocephalus, akinetic mutism, Mexico, struggles with pessimistic doctors, and more heartrending details, please read on. Forgive the long post.

I don't know whether there's anyone else on the List facing quite the same situation. I haven't seen any messages that would indicate that there are, but anyone who is dealing with a completely non-functional person probably finds themselves unable to communicate for reasons similar to mine. The situation in a (large) nutshell is this: Stel's tumor (GBM about 4 x 4.5 cm in size) has been stable since December when she had stereotactic radiosurgery (SR). Despite this, Stel has steadily lost functioning since that time, to the point that she can do nothing for herself now, except chew and swallow. I'm so deeply sad that during all these months when Stel should have been able to have some quality of life, she's had none. It's just been hospitals and nursing homes and struggles of myriad kinds.

Before SR, she had already begun to have balance problems when walking and some urinary incontinence. But cognitively she was in decent shape. Immediately after SR, her cognitive functions went way downhill. She perseverated a lot (e.g., repetitively washing her hands). She was profoundly apathetic. By late January she was confined to a wheelchair and had become incontinent of urine all the time and of feces occasionally. She had stopped feeding herself but ate well when fed. She watched a lot of TV and still had her sense of humor when watching funny movies.

During this time I asked her doctors what was going on because the tumor appeared to be stable. I got no answers that helped—only (from Henry Friedman) that we have to expect these ups and downs. I consulted a neuro-psychologist who seemed as puzzled as I was about Stel's condition and offered no help other than agreeing with me that it might be worth trying Ritalin. The oncologist prescribed a tiny dose and for a few days, Stel was much more communicative and alert. Then it seemed to stop having an effect.

In February she went into in-patient rehab to try to regain some strength, which she did. During that time, from January to March she took two rounds of CCNU and tolerated it fine. In early March she had several days of remarkable alertness and responsiveness. But it didn't last and she returned to her increasingly non-responsive state. In late March she took one round of Temodar. By early April, when she sat in the wheelchair or on the portable commode, she often would lean way to the left or right. She became spastic in her right arm, hand, and leg.

During this period, I began to research the treatment at the American Metabolic Institute in Tijuana. After more than five weeks of talking to alternative medicine researchers, AMI patients, and others, I decided the autologous vaccine treatment in conjunction with other holistic methods looked promising enough to take a shot. I took Stel to Tijuana on May 1 and we were there for seven weeks. If anyone wants to know more about the Mexican adventure, please e-mail me directly because I don't want to get into heated exchanges on the List about the subject. I'll just say here that Stel never responded to the treatment as others with GBMs whom I talked to either in person or on the phone apparently have (I met Martha and Ron Baker while we were there and she was doing, and continues to do, very well).

We found out while in Mexico that Stel had indicia of hydrocephalus on CT and MRI scans. Even though her ventricles were somewhat enlarged on MRI scans done from January on, no radiologist or other doctor here in Maryland had ever mentioned the possibility that hydrocephalus might be causing some of her problems. Stel had a few remarkable days in Mexico, especially in early June when she was trying to talk more and was laughing at jokes on TV and we all thought she was off and running. But it didn't last and in mid-June she stopped trying to talk at all. I haven't heard her voice or laugh or seen her smile since then.

I brought Stel back to Maryland thinking her surgeon could deal with the hydrocephalus. But the surgeon didn't think the hydrocephalus was that significant. She thought "white matter changes" on an MRI scan indicated radiation damage as the source of Stel's difficulties (research indicates that there's no correlation between white matter changes visible on an MRI and how an individual does clinically), which now included not being able to hold her head up when she sat in the wheelchair as well as being very sleepy and mute. Basically, the surgeon said nothing could be done about it. I ran around like a maniac getting other opinions for a few weeks. Ultimately there was a pretty even split between doctors who agreed with her surgeon and doctors who thought the hydrocephalus could be significant and that she might benefit from a shunt. In the course of this, I learned a lot about normal-pressure hydrocephalus, which is very difficult to diagnose and may or may not respond to a shunt. I also learned about akinetic mutism which can be caused by hydrocephalus as well as injury to certain brain structures. The case histories of n-p hydrocephalus and akinetic mutism in many cases track exactly what has happened to Stel over these months and describe exactly the state she's in now.

Without this personal research, I would have continued to be completely in the dark as to what may be afflicting Stel. I got no enlightenment from the doctors. Mostly, what I got—and continue to get—from them is pessimism. They see that Stel isn't talking, isn't moving, isn't following commands and, knowing her diagnosis, they basically think it's over and she ought to be in hospice. No matter that the tumor hasn't been growing for over eight months; no matter that the rest of Stel's organs are functioning fine; no matter that she still eats food she likes; no matter that there's research indicating that people in her state have been helped by shunts and/or medications like Ritalin or dopamine agonists or anti-coagulants.

She's been hospitalized twice since we got back from Mexico. The first time her steroid dose was increased to 36 mg a day. It may have helped a little. We also tried some Ritalin and an anti-Parkinsons drug, but still had a way to go in getting the dosages up to a point where the research indicated they might be helpful when the neurologist balked. (He said he didn't trust little studies from little places; I told him the study in question was from M.D. Anderson, where they now have hundreds of BT patients on Ritalin, seizure-free; when he said, "What's M.D. Anderson," I knew he wasn't the guy I wanted treating Stel.) The second hospitalization was for shunt surgery. Stel has now had the shunt 2 1/2 weeks and so far there are no signs of improvement. Her surgeon says we may have to wait weeks or months for improvement, if it ever comes, but I know she really believes Stel is suffering from radiation damage and has begun a slow deterioration from which she'll never recover. And so I sit and watch and wait and hope, as I have for months. It's a hell I could never have envisioned.

Since April 1999 when this nightmare began, I have continued to have hope that Stel can beat the odds (she's already beat the median) and that there will be life after this living hell for her and me. But so far, unfortunately, I keep striking out in my predictions of better days ahead. I've said to Stel again and again as we struggled against another obstacle in our path that it will get better, and it's only gotten worse. So I fear that I'll be wrong again, and yet I believe that where there's life, there's hope—and even though nearly everything has been taken from Stel now, she's still very much alive and I've seen the Stella I've known and loved for 31 years shining through those marvelous eyes during brief, treasured moments when we can make eye contact. The roller coaster ride continues—hopes up, hopes dashed to the ground—watching, waiting, envisioning a day when I'll see her smile again, hear her say "Kate," when I can watch her yet enjoy some of her life while she still has it.

Thanks for reading this. I'll welcome your thoughts, questions, suggestions, experiences, wisdom. Kay

Thu Sep 14 2000 10:28 PM

June, Thanks for your message. I'm interested to know that your daughter has benefited from bromocriptine. What is her dosage? Did she respond to the drug right away or did it take some time to get to the right amount? While Stel was in the hospital in July I persuaded the neurologist to try it, but we never got near the dosage—100-110 mg a day—of the medication that the patients in the studies I had seen responded to. I'm now waiting a few weeks to see whether we get any response to the shunt, but I definitely intend to pursue bromocriptine and other dopamine agonists I've read about, as well as some other drugs, further. I'm not about to give up when I know there are people in Stel's situation who have been helped. All the best to you and Jennifer, Kay

Thu Sep 14 2000 11:26 PM

Dear Kay, I want you to know that my heart is broken with yours. Your BT journey with Stel has been hell. HELL! You have done everything for her and nothing has seemed to work. You have tried so hard. Thank you for sharing your journey. As I told someone last week, if we as caregivers could eat arsenic and old lace and that would make our loved ones better, we'd do it. I think you've gone that extra mile! My thoughts and prayers remain with you and your beloved Stel. Janet

Fri Sep 15 2000 8:56 AM

Dear Melinda, Re Mexico: We had great hopes for the Mexico treatment, given the experiences of some other BT patients there, and it's been a bitter disappointment that it didn't seem to work for Stel, although it's impossible to know if it's had something to do with keeping the tumor stable this long. My next effort is going to be to get Stel to Duke so she can have a comprehensive assessment by doctors from different disciplines who specialize in brain tumors. I'm fed up with the doctors here and want to get her to a place with a more positive atmosphere and with doctors who can look her over completely and maybe help her have some quality of life. I hope to be able to get her there in October. Thanks so much for your kind words and thoughts. I'm going to keep on keeping on. Best, Kay

Fri Sep 15 2000 11:57 AM

Dear Kay, I am so sorry and can certainly sympathize with your pain. My boy, too, has not been himself for a long time. He is so sleepy. We tried Ritalin but it made him wild and hostile. It was a bad trip for him. We have thought we saw some improvement with Carbo Dopa (sp?) and Requip. These things mainly help muscle function. We were anxious to start Provigil as soon as we got the Effexor regulated. Then, of course, this last seizure episode set us back. Our doctor at Duke has also mentioned that he would like to try Aricept for memory. I know they are all drugs and I would so like something else, but I often feel trapped with no choice. I hope the very best for you and your Stel. I, too, am in sad wonder over this awful event that changed our lives so tremendously. Pat

Sat Sep 16 2000 5:30 AM

Pat, Thanks so much for your message. I'd really appreciate having a little more information about your son's regimen. What doctor at Duke is supervising the meds? I'm thinking seriously of getting Stel down to Duke in the next few weeks so she can be assessed globally by doctors who specialize in BTs. (I'll have to work it out with Henry Friedman to get her into the hospital there because I can't handle her by myself on an out-patient basis.) Re the meds: I haven't heard of Requip and I don't know Effexor. Re Provigil and Aricept, when I talked to the researcher at M.D. Anderson, she said they use Provigil for patients who can't take Ritalin. She also said they gave one patient Aricept in addition to Ritalin and it really helped. I hope so much that the meds work to help your son more. And I pray they'll help Stel when I can get her on them. Thanks, Kay

Sat Sep 16 2000 6:20 AM

Dear Charles, The shunt has been in going on three weeks now and there's still no sign of any positive response. If anything, Stel seems more sleepy than she was for several days before the surgery. Mostly she sleeps or stares off in space. I'm grateful when I can get eye contact with her. The doctor took the stitches out last Monday and set the shunt pressure a little lower. We're supposed to go back in a month. If at that time things are no better, I'm going to move heaven and earth to get Stel into the hospital at Duke, where doctors who deal only with brain tumors can do a comprehensive assessment of her and maybe come up with some ideas to help her. She's just not getting the attention she needs here. Thanks for staying in touch. Kay

Sat Sep 16 2000 6:23 AM

Carole, Would you order a book from Amazon called "A New Approach to Epilepsy" by Adrienne Richard and Joel Reiter, M.D.? Also, keep a look out for more books, articles, etc. about brain regeneration. Thanks, Kay

Sat Sep 16 2000 1:28 PM

Kay, Dr. Forman [at Duke], who is a neuro-psychiatrist, helps us with the medicines. He is supposed to be exceptionally good at this and he is one of the first ones who tried to talk to John and talks long with us. He is very open to new ideas and yet seems conservatively interested in the patient's well being. Dr. Renee Dunn was the neuro-psychiatrist who referred us to Dr. Forman, as medicines were his specialty. They are both close there with Henry Friedman. He told us to call him any time and he works with our neurologist here. As for the meds: Effexor is an anti-depressant. Requip is a sort of catalyst for Carbo Dopa (Alzheimer or Parkinson drugs for motor facilitation.) I am glad to hear of M.D. Anderson's use of these. I will have to get back to you on the regimen and its effectiveness as John was just beginning these and he had the seizures and so they were stopped. They are sure the seizures were not from the drugs. He is now back on the Zoloft, Carbo Dopa, newly on Dilantin and back up to 40 mg of Decadron a day but will be tapered down to 2.5 again in a month. I will be in touch. I wish you a miracle!! Pat

Sat Sep 16 2000 7:08 PM

[To BT List]: This is a crazy post but I feel that only you people will understand. My wife has really gone down hill in the last few months. Today was her MRI and I was almost positive it would show growth, but it didn't. I should be happy and I am but I almost wanted to hear that it was something that we could operate on or do chemo for. Instead, the doctor told us it was damage from the radiation two years ago. He couldn't tell me if it would be worse or better or if there was anything we could do about it. I feel so frustrated. Jean's tumor was so huge that I know we didn't have any choice when it came to radiation and I know they warned us but I had no idea that the treatment would be about as bad as the disease. Can anyone tell me what kind of doctor you would go to to help a person improve the effects of radiation? I promised my wife I will do anything in my power to help improve her quality of life. I've talked to a physical therapist about the muscle weakness and 45-degree angle of walking, but she also needs help with her cognitive skills and her lack of initiative. Thanks, George

Sat Sep 16 2000 9:54 PM

George, I'm facing the same possibility with my partner Stel. Even though her tumor is stable, she has progressively lost functioning. This may be due to radiation damage, some of the doctors say. It looks like a case of if the tumor doesn't get you, the treatment will. Are the doctors recommending anything for your wife? There's research on anti-Parkinson's drugs and some others that have helped some people. My problem is finding doctors here in the D.C. area who are willing to go with the research and try things, and I think I'm going to try to take Stel to Duke before long so she can get the kind of attention she needs.

As to doctors who could help, I think a neuro-psychiatrist would be the first choice. If you can't find one, look for a neuro-psychologist, who may work with a psychiatrist who can prescribe drugs. Psycho-pharmacologists or neurologists can also do this. If you're near a significant brain tumor center, you should have luck in finding a doctor versed in this. If not, it's more difficult. Let me know how things are going for you. Kay

Sun Sep 17 2000 1:35 PM

Dear Heather, I don't understand why the doctor is saying it's time for hospice for your mother, and why she can't try Temodar or something else. I'm afraid I've found the doctors (and sometimes friends) much too quick to talk about hospice. I just think when we're dealing with a disease that plays tricks with people's minds, it's wise to be very careful about deciding that the end game has come. I also know that doctors and scientists know very little about adult brain regeneration after radiation damage. Only fifteen years ago they thought the adult brain couldn't regenerate at all. Now they know that's not true, but they don't know how much it can regenerate and how fast.

Patients suffering from radiation damage or hydrocephalus or other things can appear to be on their last leg, but there are things that can help many of them—shunts, medications like Ritalin or anti-Parkinson's drugs. As we all know, this is a tricky disease. For myself, I'm not about to count Stel out until I see that there's no stopping that tumor. Right now it's been stopped more than eight months. And all her other internal organs are functioning perfectly. She still discriminates in the food she eats and still wants to eat—not as much as she would ordinarily, but it's clear she's still interested in food.

As nice as it would be to have the help of hospice care and as difficult as it is to struggle along with the minimal home health care the insurance company will pay for otherwise, I'm not going to give up hope that Stel can get better if she gets the right treatment, and I'm going to move heaven and earth to get it. I couldn't do that if I said yes to hospice. I don't know what your mother's situation is, and you have to make the best decision you can in light of all the circumstances, but I would caution against opting for hospice just because she may be suffering from radiation damage. All the best to you, Kay

Sun Sep 17 2000 6:22 PM

Dear Kay, I'm new to this group. My wife has been on Temodar since last October. Her radiologist had told us that no chemotherapy was really available for brain tumors, so we thanked him for the information and went home. Later I read in Judy's chart that "the patient has elected to forgo chemotherapy, a decision which is quite understandable." This doctor also told us to get ready for hospice two summers ago. I wonder how much less Judy would be disabled if this doctor had told us the truth about chemo and not decided for Judy that Judy didn't want to live any more. Frank

Sun Sep 17 2000 7:45 PM

Dear Kay, I can't offer a lot of practical advice, only that three months ago the doctor was prepared to stop treating my sister. I didn't accept this and showed him the results of my research and we were lucky he agreed to try what I was suggesting. I don't know if the treatment is working. I can only say my sister has had three months of much better quality of life. Previously I thought we had reached the beginning of the end, although she had not reached the stage Stel has. My point is, you are right to keep on fighting for what you believe to be the best and keep on til you find a doctor who is prepared to support you. I've seen my sister smile again when I was beginning to think I wouldn't. I hope and pray you have some success and prove all the medics wrong. Janice

Sun Sep 17 2000 10:34 PM

Frank, It's amazing the fiction you can read in charts, isn't it? The doctor's reports I've read are replete with errors, and outright lies in at least one case. Glad you didn't send Judy to hospice two years ago. Kay

Sun Sep 17 2000 10:37 PM

Janice, Thanks so much for your message. To see Stel smile again would be a wonderful gift. I'd like to know more about the treatment your doctor agreed to try. Kay

Mon Sep 18 2000 12:03 PM

Dear List: I had a similar experience. After only one week of radiation, the neurologist told me point blank that there was NO HOPE for my husband and I should consider hospice. When I questioned how he could be so certain Richard was dying, he acted as if I were a stupid woman not quite comprehending the severity of my husband's condition. The neurologist also told me that the condition that Richard was in at the time—completely paralyzed, lethargic, in coma-like state—was the best condition that I would see him and his symptoms would only worsen until he died. Divine Intervention, however, gave me the strength to tell the neurologist he was "full of—it (rhymes with hit)."

Seven months later, Richard is alive and enjoying a good quality of life. He has some minor deficits—but, hey, he is alive. He leads an active and full social life, and we are now planning a trip to Europe. I get shivers whenever I think back to that awful day when the neurologist offered me no hope. I also had to fight with the hospital social worker, who working under the neurologist's report, kept sending hospice folks to get me to take Richard home to let him die in peace. You should have seen the look on her face when she saw Richard walking!!! The moral of the story—doctors don't know everything. Get rid of the doctors who offer nothing but a death sentence. Lisa

Mon Sep 18 2000 8:18 PM

Lisa, Your message about Richard lifts my spirit as I watch and wait day by day hoping to see Stel come out of a state similar to the one he was in. Please give me more details about what brought about his recovery. Thanks, Kay

Mon Sep 18 2000 9:32 PM

Hi, Does anyone know of any treatment to reverse dementia caused by radiation necrosis? (Steve's symptoms are memory loss, confusion, paranoia—helped by Risperdal—gait problems, muscle weakness, urinary incontinence.) Thank you, Phyllis

Tue Sep 19 2000 5:08 AM

Phyllis, Most doctors will say there's nothing. But there are published studies on some drugs that have helped: Ritalin, Provigil, anti-Parkinsons meds like bromocriptine and others, anti-depressants, and anti-coagulants. Anti-Alzheimer's meds are also being used in some cases. I'm facing a similar situation and haven't found it easy to find a local doctor who is up on the research or willing to try these things very much. I'm going to try to get my partner Stel into the hospital at Duke for a comprehensive assessment and treatment plan that will include some of these meds. Another person on the list just gave me the name of the neuro-psychiatrist there, Leslie Forman, who specializes in medications and is treating her son with some of them now. The other thing I'm looking into is hyperbaric oxygen treatment, which is used to treat radiation necrosis or damage. I know of clinics in California, Florida, and Maryland, and some hospitals have the machines, although they may use them for restricted purposes. You mentioned your husband is being helped by Risperdal. Can you tell me how it's helping him? How long has he been taking it and at what dosage? What doctor prescribed it? All the best, Kay

Tue Sep 19 2000 4:48 PM

Dear Mary, I'm so sorry to hear about your sister, but grateful it was a peaceful ending. I know how painful her loss must be for you. Stel's fight continues. Since her shunt surgery three weeks ago, she's been so sleepy that we're having a CT scan done tomorrow to see if there's bleeding going on, and now she's got a temperature, which may indicate infection. Waiting for lab results. I'm making plans to get her down to Duke by ambulance soon so she can have a comprehensive evaluation and treatment plan. I send you my kindest thoughts and hopes for future happiness. Kay

Tue Sep 19 2000 5:14 PM

Lisa, Thanks very much for your response. Richard's story is inspiring. I'd be interested to know where you live and who Richard's doctor is. I take it he hasn't had any bad side effects from the Thalidomide—i.e., making him even more lethargic than he already was. I hope one day to have a similar story to tell about Stel. How wonderful it would be to see her open her eyes and try to talk or smile. Again, thanks. Kay

Tue Sep 19 2000 8:37 PM

Dear Mona, I'm deeply touched by your message. You're right. I do love Stel beyond all words. And I still believe she can be a survivor if we can find the right treatment to help her start functioning again. I've been very depressed all day because she was sleeping and sleeping and then tonight she suddenly held her head up straight for several minutes, something she hasn't done in quite a while, and hope sprang up in my heart once again. Tomorrow I have to get her to the hospital for a CT scan to rule out (I hope) any bleeding from the shunt surgery as the reason for her sleepiness. Oh, please, please, please let Stella come back one of these days!! Thank you. It's so kind of you to think of us. Kay

Tue Sep 19 2000 9:33 PM

Dr. Friedman, You should receive Stel's latest MRI done on September 11th tomorrow. The tumor remains stable, as it has since last December.

I just talked to Dr. Raj [oncologist] who advised me that you had indicated there is no way you can see Stel as an in-patient at Duke. I am deeply distressed because I feel sure that the only chance she has for getting better and having some quality of life is for her to get the kind of comprehensive attention she could get there from doctors in different disciplines who specialize in brain tumors. She just can't get that here. I've gone crazy trying to find doctors who aren't completely pessimistic, who are well-versed enough in the latest research and open to trying things they haven't tried before, and who will communicate with other doctors, and I just feel pretty certain that all Stel will continue to get is fragmented attention and ad hoc treatment. I had so much hope that at Duke she could get the attention she needs now if she is to have the possibility of regaining some of her functioning, and I just don't know what to do at this point.

It makes no sense to me that Stel's tumor has been stable all this time and yet she can't function. All she can do is chew and swallow on her own—and she definitely still does that and discriminates in the food she eats. I could understand her being in this shape if we were in the end game, but that's not the case. All of her internal organs are operating fine. I know she understands me when we make eye contact and I talk to her. She's not in any pain. But she's trapped in this state of akinetic mutism. I've read enough (and talked to researchers enough) to know that some people in this state have been helped by a variety of medications—not only Ritalin, but Provigil, Aricept, Cogentin, Prolopa, L-Dopa and others. I know that shunts have helped in some cases, too, but according to her surgeon we may not know for weeks or months if the shunt she placed three weeks ago is going to have a positive effect.

I don't want to leave any stone unturned in trying to help Stel. I have much more confidence that all possibilities will be considered at Duke than I do that it will happen here. Stel is not in an unstable condition. She simply can't function and I can't handle her by myself. If I brought her down there in an ambulance, could someone at Duke help me find a way to manage her as an out-patient? In other words, could I get help in finding accommodations that would be suitable for a handicapped person, in hiring a nurse or aide to assist me, in arranging for ambulance transportation back and forth? I've already talked to Stacy there and know Duke doesn't provide any facilities itself. Would you see Stel at the clinic if she came in an ambulance and could you arrange to have her assessed by neuro-oncology, neuro-psychiatry, neuro-psychology, neurosurgery, neurology and whatever else in a few days? Could the team come up with a comprehensive treatment plan for her (and perhaps some ideas of doctors in this area who might work with doctors at Duke)? I'd be especially interested in having Dr. Forman see her and make some recommendations. Also, I know that Dr. A. Friedman along with Drs. Radtke and Massey of Neurology at Duke were involved in a heparin/warfarin study and I'd like their input.

I don't want to take up more of your time with a longer message. If it would be helpful, I can fax you a chronology of what's happened with Stel over the past eight months and where she is now. Please let me know if you want me to send such a summary. I'd appreciate talking to you in the next few days. You can reach me at 301-657-3713 most of the time. If you prefer, I can page you. All I can say at this point is please help me try in every possible way to help Stel. She needs (and I need) the hope that Duke offers instead of the hopelessness that is too often served up by doctors who don't know what surprises are possible in the brain tumor universe. Thanks, Kay

Tue Sep 19 2000 9:40 PM

Kay, I know the big list is not really into "alternative meds" but I can't help but wonder if this Poly-MVA stuff may be worth trying. What do you know about it? Mona

Tue Sep 19 2000 9:48 PM

Mona, Stel has been taking Poly-MVA since May when we went to Mexico for a vaccine treatment. Unfortunately, I can't say that either it or the vaccine have done for Stel what they appear to have done for others. On the other hand, her tumor has remained stable throughout all these months when she hasn't been on any other treatment, so maybe that's due to the Poly and/or the vaccine. I'm continuing to give her the Poly because she's not on anything else now and I hope with every MRI to see a change I can attribute to it. I'm reluctantly probably going to try to get her back on a chemo soon, but Dr. Friedman wanted to wait a bit to see how she responds, if she does, to the shunt she recently had placed. I feel like I'm playing Russian roulette with Stel's life. It's all nerve-wracking. All the best, Kay

Wed Sep 20 2000 10:15 AM

Dear Peter, The days are very hard to get through. No signs yet of any improvement. (She does seem to be moving her head a little more than she has, but whether that means anything or will lead anywhere else, god knows.) In fact, Stel has been sleeping much more than she was, so I called the surgeon about that. She wanted to get a CT scan and I've got to get Stel over to the hospital this afternoon for that—not an easy task. If it shows bleeding, of course, that will mean more surgery. Then yesterday the visiting nurse found she had a fever of 102. So urine and blood tests are being done for that. It's also possible that's related to the shunt. As of now, I have no idea what the afternoon will hold. Also, I had hoped to make arrangements to take Stel down to Duke by ambulance for a comprehensive evaluation, but I just found out yesterday that Duke won't take her as an inpatient—too many people clamoring for too few beds—and I don't know if there's any way I can manage to deal with her there as an out-patient. Unbelievably, the university doesn't make any provisions for accommodations or transportation for people who aren't able to get around. So I'm fretting about what I can do this morning. The oncologist was going to call Johns Hopkins to see what, if anything, they can do, but I have my doubts they'll offer anything more and I also have my doubts they are into the kinds of medications I want to try. They're more conservative than Duke.

She needs doctors from different disciplines to look at her from different angles. Getting that here in Bethesda appears to be impossible. What I'd give to be living in L.A. I think we might have been able to help Stel much earlier if I'd had doctors who had some knowledge about what was happening to her back in January-February when I was asking the doctors here. Wish I had better news. I'll let you know the upshot of our hospital trek today. Kay

Wed Sep 20 2000 8:00 PM

[To BT List]: Teresa is having trouble with mucas in the back of her throat. We were having trouble suctioning it out and even when we got it out, it quickly returned. As she breathed, we could hear it. Hospice didn't give us much help with this. But we found a nurse who really knows her stuff and she showed us how to suction through the nose. It is gross, but when you can't get to it from the mouth, it works. We are also using a transderm patch on Teresa. It helped a lot. She was being suctioned about every half hour before the patch; now it is like every four hours or so. It isn't indicated for that—it is for seasickness—but the nurse suggested it, and it seems to help. One patch every three days. Ben

Wed Sep 20 2000 8:45 PM

Ben, Is the patch something you just buy in the drug store? Where do you put it and how does it work to clear the mucus? I've been wondering what to do about this for Stel. Kay

Thu Sep 21 2000 5:59 AM

Dear Peter, The CT scan showed a little bit of blood accumulation, but the doctor didn't think it is enough to cause Stel to be so sleepy. However, it is enough to indicate that the pressure can't be set any lower. So if the shunt is going to work, it will have to work at this pressure. Doctor said sleepiness is probably part of "inexorable neurologic decline." It's always such an upper to talk to her. Stel does have a urinary tract infection, which probably accounts for the fever. I'm hoping this may have caused some of her sleepiness. Somehow I've got to get her under the care of a doctor who can and will administer medications that might help her. That's it for now. Love, Kay

Thu Sep 21 2000 9:18 PM

[To Kay Loveland]: The MRI shows diffuse tumor/rt damage. We have nothing to offer except the possibility that medication would help. We recommend Ritalin—ask your doc to call me—maybe we can wake her up with this. Henry [Friedman]

Fri Sep 22 2000 9:42 AM

Kay, What about doctors at NIH? They have a brain tumor center there now. They may even have some trials that would help. Barbara

Fri Sep 22 2000 10:06 AM

Barbara, I've been in touch with Dr. Howard Fine, head of the Neuro-oncology Unit there. He consulted on some questions I had, but he's not Stel's treating physician. Stel wasn't eligible for a clinical trial we discussed because she's really unable to do anything for herself. I don't think she'd be accepted in any trial now. NIH is great if you can take advantage of the trials, but if you can't, I don't get the impression it's a place to go for just regular treatment. If you know anything different, please advise me. Thanks, Kay

Sat Sep 23 2000 6:21 AM

Dear Karla, I just wanted you to know how much I appreciated your calling. It means a lot in very dark days. Next week I'm mounting an intensive search for a neurologist or neuro-psychiatrist here who will try to help Stel with the medications I've read about in research articles. Love, Kay

Sun Sep 24 2000 6:43 AM

Dear Dr. Meyers, I'm writing to you again because I need your help in getting treatment for Stella with medications that may help her regain some cognitive and motor functioning. As I indicated when I contacted you in July, I was trying to work with a neurologist here in Bethesda to give Stella Ritalin. We did ultimately get her dosage up to 30 mg twice a day. As I had said in my message to you, we thought we saw a response when we began the medication at 5 mg twice a day, but it didn't seem to continue, and I couldn't note any perceptible response up to and including the 60 mg a day dosage. At that point, the neurologist balked at going any higher even though I told him of my conversation with you in which you said you have patients taking 60 mg twice a day. Did those patients evidence any response before you got them to that level?

As you know, her tumor has been stable since last December, but she's lost all functioning, except chewing and swallowing. (She's still interested in food when she's not too sleepy to make the effort.) She's very much alive but has no life. She's usually either sleeping or staring off in space—and when she stares, she sometimes appears to be seeing a vision that frightens or startles her. After a lot of consultation, I had a shunt placed at the end of August because of somewhat enlarged ventricles. The intracranial pressure has been reduced by 4 cm, from 13 to 9, but to date there's no indication that it is having any effect on her functioning (although she has moved her head several times in the last few days, a new phenomenon.)

Stella has been treated with chemo under the supervision of Dr. Henry Friedman. When I spoke to him day before yesterday about her condition, he recommended using Ritalin. I told him of our conversation about the higher dosages of Ritalin and about your anecdotal experience with adding Aricept to the mix. He thought this sounded like a possible approach but said he had no experience with using Ritalin at the higher doses or combining it with Aricept and felt it would be a good idea for me to get a recommendation from you that could be provided to her oncologist. I would like very much to try the Ritalin/Aricept combination, starting as soon as possible, if you think that makes sense. I know you said the patient you treated with the combination had radiation dementia and required 24-hour supervision. Stella is in the same situation, it appears. Would it be best for me to have the oncologist call you, or could you e-mail me a recommendation or fax it to the oncologist?

I would appreciate talking to you again and will call you. I'm at my wit's end in finding a neuro-psychiatrist, neuro-psychopharmacologist, or neurologist here to work with and wonder whether you would have suggestions of colleagues in the area I could contact. Also, more generally, can you tell me if there are BT centers in the East that are doing similar work with medications to what you're doing at M.D. Anderson? I wanted to take Stella down to Duke (by ambulance) for a comprehensive in-patient evaluation, but Dr. Friedman said that's not possible and indicated that Duke doesn't do much in the area of medications. I really believe Stella needs comprehensive attention paid to her condition and all aspects of medications (including anti-seizure—e.g., she's taking 1200 a day of Tegretol;

might she do better on another, newer, anti-seizure med?) and want to get that for her. I'd even contemplate trying to get her to Houston if you thought it would help. I don't want to leave any stone unturned in trying to help her regain some functioning. I've seen research on dopamine agonists that might be helpful. We tried a little bromocriptine along with the Ritalin last summer. She got up to 40 mg a day, but the research I've seen had patients at 100-110 mg to get a response. I don't know whether it made sense to use both of them together; it was not a decision made with any deliberation on the neurologist's part. I don't know whether you're doing work there at M.D. Anderson with these medications as well. If not, I'd appreciate any direction you may have to doctors who are working with them.

Please forgive me for taking up so much of your time with this, but I'm feeling rather desperate right now. Dr. Friedman said he hadn't seen many cases like this and from everything I've learned in the past few weeks, it does appear to me to be rather an unusual case that most doctors don't seem to know what to do with. I know it's quite possible that nothing may help Stella, but I don't plan to give up until I've tried everything that offers some hope, and being with her 24 hours a day, I know there's a person still there who's trapped inside herself and I often feel is on the verge of breaking out.

I should mention, I guess, that Stella had about seven seizures (focal; no loss of consciousness) during the year from August 1999 through July 2000. At least half of them were attributable to tumor growth, surgery, or radiosurgery. While she was taking Ritalin, she had one small focal seizure after she had been on the 60 mg a day dose for several days. Her Tegretol level was found to be quite high and the neurologist said that could have caused it with the other meds she was on. Her only med at present is Tegretol. She's had about four more small focal seizures (lasting 15-20 seconds max; no loss of consciousness) in the past few weeks—at least one of which was attributable to a low Tegretol level. She's had no seizures in the last couple of weeks. She has had EEGs during her hospital stays this summer that have not shown any on-going seizure activity. Also, right now she's not on any chemo treatment, but she may start on something again soon. Do you have patients taking the Ritalin and also chemo at the same time?

Please let me know if there's anything I need to do to engage your services as a consultant. I will be so grateful for anything you can do to help. I'll look forward to talking to you. Kay

Mon Sep 25 2000 10:11 AM

Dear Kay, It sounds like you have a pretty awful situation to deal with. I have had numerous patients that have bifrontal radiation/tumor injury that are in the same state as Stella. Unfortunately we have had little success in improving their cognitive function and motivation at that stage; our successes have mostly been with patients who are somewhat better functionally (even though, by normal control standards, they are profoundly impaired). Henry Friedman is one of the best neuro-oncologists in the nation; you can't go wrong with him. There is a neuro-psychologist in his group, Dr. Renee Dunn, who is doing (or has recently completed) a study of Aricept in brain tumor patients. There is also a wonderful support team there headed by Bebe Guill. I would suggest talking with them first, as there are no signposts along this road—we truly just treat by the seat of our pants. Dr. Dunn's e-mail is dunn0016@mc.duke.edu; Ms. Guill's e-mail: guill004@mc.duke.edu. If I can be of help, however, please let me know. Christina [Meyers]

Mon Sep 25 2000 2:08 PM

Dear Christina, Thanks for the information. I'll follow up. I assume you don't have a reference to any doctors in the Bethesda-D.C. area who could serve as a local contact. Is it your view, then, that pursuing the Ritalin-Aricept combination with Stella would be fruitless? Kay

Mon Sep 25 2000 3:37 PM

Dear Kay, I admit I would not be optimistic about improvement, but on the other hand, there is nothing to lose by trying, and certainly nothing to gain by doing nothing. I don't know of neurologists nearby you, but I'll list below board-certified neuro-psychologists (like myself) who might be helpful or know who could be. Good luck, and don't hesitate to contact me if you need any other information, or (for what it's worth), guidance. Christina.

Mon Sep 25 2000 3:44 PM

Christina, Sorry to keep pestering you, but if we wanted to start Stella in the next few days on the Ritalin/Aricept regimen, could you provide guidance to the oncologist on where to start and how to proceed? Should I ask her to call you? Thanks, Kay

Mon Sept 25 2000 4:02 PM

Kay, You're not pestering! The Aricept dose is what is prescribed for Alzheimer's patients, whatever that is (I don't know)—and I guess I would keep the Ritalin at the last dose she was on at first, since you know there are no adverse effects. Chris

Mon Sep 25 2000 4:15 PM

Christina, Thanks for responding so quickly. So it wouldn't be a problem starting Stel at 30 mg twice a day instead of starting her lower and increasing the dosage as we did initially? Re the Aricept dose, would the oncologist just ask the drug company what the prescribed dose is? Thanks also for sending the names of the doctors. I've already sent e-mails to them. I can't thank you enough. Kay

Mon Sep 25 2000 8:57 PM

Hi everyone [on BT List], Does anyone have knowledge or experience with the anti-psychotic drug Risperdal? My husband Steve started on 1/2 mg (twice/day) two mos ago for hostile, threatening behavior, and by mid-Aug was up to his present 2 mg twice daily. He's calm now, but "out of it" most of the time and sleeps twenty or more hours a day. Also has lost muscle mass and is incredibly weak. His recurrent brain mets are stable, with necrosis being blamed for his mental deterioration and peripheral vision loss, etc. MRI done 9/18 shows improvement in both, and a recent spinal tap ruled out excess hydrocephalus as the cause of sleeping and weakness. Neurosurgeon "can't understand why MRI shows improvement but Steve isn't any better."

Do you think the Risperdal is part of the problem, or do we just have to assume the surgeon's "guess" that small blood vessel rad damage and maybe nerve damage are the answer? I'm at a loss, overwhelmed by trying to figure out what's wrong and how to help him. A couple of weeks ago his onc signed hospice papers (just so I would get more assistance, I think) but told me he wouldn't be surprised if Steve's condition became chronic, with no particular prognosis as to life expectancy. I don't know whether to prepare for his passing or try to accept the idea of YEARS like this! HELP if you can. I feel like I've been getting nowhere with the docs, and it's as if they have NO CLUE what's really wrong, so they just avoid my questions. Thanks so much. I don't post often, but get a lot of helpful info from all of you on the List. I've only been going through this since June of this year. Before that, Steve was "okay," just a little forgetful and needing a daily nap. Then I guess the "long-term radiation damage" began to rear its ugly head. I am hurting every day at the loss of my best friend and dearest person to my heart. He isn't Steve any more, and the docs don't expect recovery from these mental deficits. Phyllis

Mon Sept 25 2000 10:26 PM

Dear Phyllis, I'm grieving, as you are, over the loss of my best friend and dearest person and the prospect that her condition may be chronic as well. I don't know anything about Risperdal, but I certainly wouldn't count it out since Steve has gotten worse on it. Are you saying that the MRI showed that his necrosis has improved? I didn't think that was possible. How can they tell?

I'm also going crazy looking for ways to help Stel. As I think I told you, I want to try various medications that have helped others with radiation injury. I've been in touch with several doctors today about this. And if these things don't help, I'm going to pursue hyperbaric oxygen treatment. If what is involved with Steve is small vessel damage, such treatment might be worth pursuing for him. I know it helps with repairing small blood vessels. I've had the same experience with doctors—they don't have a clue. If I hadn't done research myself, I'd still be in the dark about what may be afflicting Stel and what treatments might help. Most doctors throw up their hands, first, at GBM and then at radiation damage. Just remember that fifteen years ago scientists didn't think the adult brain could regenerate at all. But they found out it can. So they can talk all they want about how it's never going to get better, but they don't really know that.

This is a very painful situation to be in and, again, I feel like I've been sideswiped, as I did when Stel was diagnosed. I had no idea this could happen; no doctor ever mentioned anything about the possibility of permanent radiation damage except in passing, and it hit us unaware. All we can do is keep on keeping on. I'm with you in the struggle. All the best, Kay

Monday, September 25, 2000

FAX to Dr. Leslie Forman, Dept. of Psychiatry, Duke Univ. Med. Center

I learned from the mother of a patient on the Internet Brain Tumor List that you are treating him for sleepiness and other manifestations of possible radiation injury with various medications. I am seeking similar help for my partner, Stella Sandris. I'm attaching a chronology of her history.

I know from research that patients in the state she is now in have sometimes been helped with medications such as Ritalin, L-Dopa, bromocriptine, and anti-depressants. I want to obtain this treatment for Stella but have so far not been able to find doctors in the D.C. area to provide it. I have been in touch with Dr. Christina Meyers at M.D. Anderson who told me of their success with Ritalin at doses up to 120 mg a day. As you'll note on the attached chronology, in July Stella was on Ritalin, up to 60 mg a day, but there was no perceptible response. At the same time, the neurologist also tried bromocriptine—up to 40 mg a day along with the Ritalin. I don't know whether it made sense to combine these two drugs; he just tried it after I showed him the research on bromocriptine.

Dr. Henry Friedman has supervised some chemo treatment for Stella, but she is presently not being treated. He is concerned that in her condition it would harm her more. Last week he recommended that we try Ritalin. I asked about contacting you and he encouraged me to do so. What I had hoped would be possible would be to bring Stella down to Duke in an ambulance and have her receive a comprehensive evaluation as an in-patient. Dr. Friedman said that wasn't possible. I don't know whether you could do that or not. I just feel that given the unusualness of her situation, as Dr. Friedman said (tumor stable for so many months but she's unable to function at all), and its severity, that she would benefit most from an in-patient assessment. I could try to bring her down on an out-patient basis, but it's much more difficult for me to deal with her that way. I would need Duke's help to arrange manageable accommodations, assistance, and transportation.

I really don't know what to do at this point. I want to get Stella started on some treatment for her condition as soon as possible. If there is a doctor in this area with whom you have worked or who you know is knowledgeable about these medications, I'd appreciate your advising me. I would hope to have a local doctor who would consult with you, as the local oncologist consults with Dr. Friedman. As you may be able to tell, I'm at my wit's end in trying to deal with this problem and will deeply appreciate any help and advice you can give me. I anxiously await hearing from you. Sincerely, Kay Loveland

Tue Sep 26 2000 2:10 PM

Dear Dr. Burnett, At Dr. Cifu's suggestion, I telephoned you today to talk with you about whether it makes sense for me to try to bring Stella Sandris to Richmond for evaluation and treatment there. I forwarded to you my e-mail outlining her condition. She is unable to do anything for herself and because of the difficulty that causes in moving her, I would have to transport her by ambulance. I am seeking pharmacologic treatment for her with medications such as L-Dopa and other dopamine agonists; Ritalin or Provigil; Aricept, and other drugs that have been reported in research studies as sometimes effective for brain tumor patients in Stella's situation. If this is an option at the Center, then I would be interested in having her evaluated there. Consequently, I would very much appreciate talking to you as soon as possible about treatment options at the Center. I look forward to hearing from you at your earliest convenience. Thanks, Kay Loveland

Tue Sep 26 2000 2:45 PM

Dear Jeanne [Wallace], I know you've been moving so I waited to forward these messages to you until now. I'm sending them to bring you up to date on what's happening with Stel. It's been a heartbreaking time. Needless to say, it's tremendously lonely for me and I'm simply going through hell. I can't even hear my beloved's voice any longer. I've had no help from the doctors here in trying to figure out what was happening with her, so I had to do my own research. Now I'm desperately looking for the right doctors who might be able to help her pharmacologically. They're few and far between, and extremely sparse in this area. If, as it appears more and more, we are dealing with delayed radiation injury, treatment options are pretty limited, but I intend to pursue every possible one if I can find the doctors to do it. Dr. Rubio of AMI has told me some things to give Stel for brain regeneration. She's also getting Poly-MVA. I'm still giving her some of the supplements you had recommended. If you have any suggestions or recommendations for things to help with brain regeneration, or of doctors I should contact, please let me know. Many thanks, Kay

Tue Sep 26 2000 4:46 PM

Dear Phyllis, You wrote: <It seems everyone (medical people, including hospice), just want me to accept things as they are and be grateful that he's sleeping peacefully with no pain. If I could be sure nothing else can be done for him, I would probably accept that, but still be mad as hell that we were blindsided about the rad damage—and torn in pieces in a way I never would have expected in a million years. Through all other illnesses and stressors, you as a loving couple can manage to cope because you have each other to lean on, talk to, commiserate with. Now I have to do everything for us AND cope with the strain by myself, except for the kindness of friends and children, and strangers like you. I miss

Steve. Feels like I will have to go through the grieving process twice—now and when he's gone. The hyperbaric oxygen sounded good to me when I read about it recently, but every time I bring up anything to his onc, he seems to pooh-pooh it (the damage is done, can't be fixed, his condition is frail, etc.). My heart breaks for him and I don't want him to suffer like this, being lost inside his confused head. Do you understand?>

I understand all too well. Yes, everyone seems to think we should give up our loved one's lives so easily. Just throw up our hands and say there's nothing to be done. As for the rad damage, blindsided is right. I thought we were fighting a tumor and was happy when we stopped it in its tracks. Little did we know that the treatment would become more of a menace than the tumor in these months. As you say, it's so heartbreaking, and much too much for one person to bear. I'm grieving every day while I'm caring for Stel. I'm still grateful I can hold her, tell her I love her, but god is it lonely. I just break down sometimes and wail like a banshee. I miss her and her smile and her voice so much. My heart aches for you and Steve and for Stel and me. Kay

Tue Sep 26 2000 5:00 PM

Dear Kay, I assume the dosing of Aricept is in the PDR and package insert. I don't see any reason to start at a lower Ritalin dose, since that wasn't effective anyway. Christina
[Meyers]

Wed Sep 27 2000 9:10 PM

Christina, I forgot to ask: If we start the Ritalin/Aricept combo, would we expect to see an immediate response, if there is going to be one, or would it take a few days/weeks? In other words, how long should we stay at the same dosage before going up if we don't see a response? Can the Aricept dosage be raised as well as the Ritalin? Is 60 mg twice a day still your high point with Ritalin? Also, are a lot of your patients on chemo treatment at the same time? Finally, I take it you don't work with dopamine agonists and other drugs that have been used. Any suggestion of doctors/centers who do? Sorry. My one question turned into twenty. Kay

Wed Sep 27 2000 9:45 PM

Dear Phyllis, Sorry I didn't respond sooner. It's been one of those days—as they all are. I had to get Stel to the hospital this afternoon. She has two infections—urinary tract and blood—and so far they haven't responded to the antibiotics she's been given. She kept getting fever spikes, so the doctor said get her to the hospital. I just came home from there. I hate coming to an empty apartment and empty bed and leaving Stel there in that hospital room. This is the third time since July she's been in the hospital for one thing or another. It's wearing me down.

Re: your questions: <If the blood vessels can't convey oxygen to parts of the brain, then you must have brain tissue death as a result, right?> I don't know that it would initially be brain tissue death. Could be just damage, which I understand can be greatly helped with hyperbaric oxygen. Also, I think I mentioned previously the Parkinson's drugs that have been helpful to some patients in Steve's condition. The problem is finding a doctor to prescribe them. I'm actively working on that now. I should also mention that I give Stel liquid amino acids, lecithin, and a supplement called Phosphatidycholine Concentrate (or PhosChol) by American Lecithin Company. These are all supposed to help with brain regeneration. <How are you finding ways to cope?> I cry and scream whenever I just can't bear it any more. Otherwise, I just keep on keeping on because I have to. I figure there'll be plenty of time to fall apart if we don't win this war. <Because it's not their spouse, and because they have a life to go home to after seeing his sad condition, they can't understand that caring for my dearest companion 24/7 stresses me to the end of my ability to cope sometimes.> Yes, we can't leave the sadness and return to the mundane world. Whenever I'm out shopping and the clerk says, "Have a nice day," I want to say, "If you only knew." <Do you forget to eat sometimes also?> Not usually. I feed myself before Stel if I can so I won't get too busy and forget it, because I know I'm going to be no good if I don't eat and sleep, which I usually manage to do.

<Yesterday I went to the beach and I thought this will be peaceful and relaxing. WRONG! I was forgetting that Steve and I have a lot of memories that include beaches. What on earth was I thinking? I just sat there and cried on the beach, then drove home.> I know. When I go out to places Stel and I have been together or know she would like to go, I can hardly bear it. I get so sad and just want to get home where I can see her and touch her and talk to her. People keep saying it'll do you good to get out, but it just intensifies the sense of loss. I don't know how I'll ever take the trips she and I wanted to take without feeling that aching pain. Again, I know there'll be plenty of time to feel that way if we lose the struggle; I don't know how much time I have to be with Stel, whatever her condition, and I want all of those precious moments. <I know everyone says caregivers have to do

things they enjoy or we'll burn out, but it's hard to defocus from Steve. Most of my time out of the house has to be spent running errands.> That's how I spend my "free" time, but I can't imagine enjoying myself while I know Stel is lying in bed unable to move. We always loved doing things together; if I'm out doing something I know she would enjoy (and we always liked to do the same kinds of things), I just get sadder and sadder. Maybe some people can divorce themselves from the situation, but I'm not one of them. I've never been a person who felt a great need to have my own "space." I enjoyed being with Stel and doing things with her.

<Someone I spoke to today about this issue said I sort of have to reinvent my life. I guess that may be true, but I don't want to leave Steve behind. I miss him a lot, as you do Stel.> There'll be plenty of time for reinventing. I want to cherish Stel as long as I have her. <Today, though, he called for me twice, just to tell me "I love you"! I was thrilled and told him that was better than a million dollars.> To hear Stel tell me she loves me would be the thrill of a lifetime now. I get excited when we just have a moment of eye contact, which has been practically non-existent the last few days. She spoke her last word to me on June 14th. However, she did give me some wonderful kisses for several days after that, and then that stopped, too. I have to cling to those memories now and hope she proves the doctors wrong and one day speaks and smiles and kisses again. Must get to bed. Days at the hospital are very tiring. Thanks for your messages, too. It helps to know there's someone who truly understands—but I'm sorry it has to be that way, for all of us. Love, Kay

Wednesday, September 27, 2000
FAX to Dr. Raj

I want to touch base with you about the following: (1) Dr. Friedman recommended trying Ritalin. I told him we had tried it to some extent in July-August but had never taken the dose as high as 120 mg a day, which Dr. Meyers said they have done with many patients. I also told him that she was using Aricept along with Ritalin for a particularly unresponsive patient and had had good results and said I would like to do that with Stel. He said that sounded okay but he knows very little about this area and we should get a recommendation from Dr. Meyers. I've been in touch with Dr. Meyers and she agreed it is worth trying the combination with Stel. She thought we could start with the 30 mg twice a day dose of Ritalin Stel was taking up until her shunt surgery. She said the dose of Aricept should be whatever is recommended in the PDR or package insert. Since

I've not yet found a neuro-psychiatrist or neurologist to deal with this aspect of Stel's medications, I'd appreciate it if you would write these prescriptions so that once Stel's infections are under control, she could begin taking them.

(2) Dr. Friedman continues to be of the view that we shouldn't put Stel on any chemo treatment right now because it might make things worse. I'm not so sure about this. Things couldn't get much worse. I've read of people on the BT List who were in as bad or worse condition (practically comatose) who received various chemo treatments and actually improved. If we were fortunate enough to get some shrinkage of the tumor, it seems to me that could help Stel. At any rate, I'm getting worried about not having her on any treatment for so many months. What is your thought about it? I'm wondering about using CCNU, which Stel tolerated well in December-February, maybe in combination with Accutane, which seems pretty mild in its side effects. Stel has another MRI scheduled for October 24th when we do another shunt follow-up with Dr. Neiman. I don't think I'd want to wait any later than that to get going on something again if at all possible.

(3) As you know, I gave Chris the names of two neuro-psychiatrists at Johns Hopkins and would be interested to know what they are doing, if anything, with medications for BT patients.

I'd like to talk to you about these matters and will appreciate your calling me as soon as you can. Thanks, Kay

Fri Sep 29 2000 6:53 AM

Dear Phyllis, You wrote: <The nurse explained that it's almost impossible to get Steve to an appointment in his frail, exhausted condition.> I'm beside myself with trying to figure out how to get Stel seen by a neurologist or neuro-psychiatrist here so I can get a local doctor to help administer the medications I want to try with her. I have to take her by ambulance, which costs a bundle every time I do it, and trying to explain that to a new doctor's office is a trial. I just got the name of a neurologist whose office is half a block from our building, so I thought at least that would be easy, but when I think about it, I don't know how I'll do it. I'm afraid Stel can't even sit up in the wheelchair long enough for me to wheel her there, and the wheeling is not over the smoothest terrain. I'm thinking it would be so easy for the doctor to come to our apartment, but you know that's a pipedream, although I'll broach it. Actually, I told her oncologist I'd like him to come to the hospital while Stel is there to see her and she said she'd call him, but now I'll have to call her to see if she got him and if he's coming and, of course, if he is, there's no telling when, so I have to stay in the room constantly if I want to have any chance of talking to him when and if he comes. It's just crazy that patients who are unable to get to a doctor's office really can't get the care they need.

I spoke to the neuro-psychiatrist at Duke yesterday. He was wonderful and our talk convinced me I'm right, that if Stel has any hope of improving with the medications, she has to have the attention of doctors at a BT center like Duke. He knows all the meds and is willing to consider all the possibilities. Of course, the crazy part here, too, is that a patient who so desperately needs to be there can't be admitted as an in-patient (not enough beds) and so I have to find some way to cope with the situation on an out-patient basis. The doctor told me the social worker there would help me, but I've already talked with her and know there's nothing special provided by Duke to help patients in Stel's situation. You'd think these world-renowned centers would make some provision for patients who can't do things for themselves, but they don't—or at least Duke doesn't. At Duke There Is Hope (their motto) if you're able to get there on your own. But somehow I'm going to get her there for an evaluation because it's imperative. I had called an ambulance service a couple of weeks ago to see if they could drive her down to Duke (it's five hours) and they said they could and quoted me a price substantially cheaper than the air ambulance, so I felt at least I had an option. Yesterday I called them again to confirm the information I had and they told me they stopped doing long-distance service two weeks ago (that was when I called them). I couldn't believe it—another hurdle thrown in my path. I'll check a few other ambulance services to see if anyone else will do it, but it looks likely that I'll have to fly her down there for considerable dollars. But the possibility that she may regain some life is far more important. I'm tearing my hair out and crying my eyes out over all this.

<It's never 'over til it's over,' and miracles sometimes happen (though I'm a realist when faced with hard facts), so it's always possible that something good may happen and Steve will 'graduate' from hospice, as the nurse says.> Yes, as I said, they really don't know much of anything about adult brain regeneration. <I was all in a turmoil this afternoon because I had to begin the process with a Medicaid lawyer of spousal assessment of our assets (on the advice of the hospice social worker). It may never be an issue, but if Steve went so far downhill that I had to have 24-hour nursing care at some point, it would leave me penniless within a very short time. I WANT to keep him home, and would rather pay a nurse full-

time than go the nursing home route. He would want to be home, too. I want him as comfortable as he can possibly be under the circumstances.> I haven't yet looked into Medicaid because I knew Stel had substantially more than the $2,000 she's allowed to qualify, but I need to do that. Will Medicaid pay for 24-hour nursing care at home? I know it would pay for a nursing home, but like you, I will not put Stel in one. We've already been there three times for rehab and other reasons and I won't subject her to that long term. I want her with me. So if Medicaid would help with at least some of the nursing bill, that would be worth my doing whatever has to be done to qualify her.

<Tomorrow is our 12th anniversary, and it's already too sad to deal with. His kids are going to make some kind of occasion of it (that's how much they care!), but today when I read my journal entry of our wedding day on the beach, he wasn't responding at all. I'll try to be upbeat for their sakes, but doubt that it will reach the inner recesses of Steve's brain.> I know. It's so painful when you try to remember something with them and they clearly aren't with you. I had these romantic notions that after 31 years of incredible closeness, we'd always have some way of communicating or relating in a special way, but that's not the case. I know Stel knows I'm there; I can feel that; but otherwise she's a sphinx. It's too painful for words. <I hope things improve and you can bring Stel home soon.> Yes. Being at the hospital is very hard on me—running back and forth; being there constantly in order to try to see the doctors. And I can't relate to Stel there on even the minimal level I do at home. I hope we'll be back "home" (this apartment is just a place where illness is happening; we shared no good times here) by early next week and that I can begin planning in earnest to get her to Duke. (And that I will be able to "hire" a good doctor here to work with the doctors at Duke.) I hope your wedding anniversary yields some moments of happiness and solace, despite the tragedy of the situation. Kay

Fri Sep 29 2000 6:58 AM

Carole, Yes, I saw the article on "consciousness." It is certainly my approach to Stel—talking to her, touching her, playing music she knows by heart, etc. It's also the reason I got so mad when doctors talked over her to me about hospice, etc. I doubt the article would be of any use to the doctors, particularly since they seem to pay no attention to any information I give them, but it's useful to me to know it. Thanks, Kay

Fri Sep 29 2000 11:12 AM

Dear Kay, I'm not sure how long the response to Aricept takes; that should be in the PDR. Ditto raising the dose. We have had one person on 80 mg twice a day of Ritalin who had progressive radiation injury, but really no dose made any difference at that point. Many of our patients are on active chemo treatment during stimulant therapy. We are also in the process of conducting trials of modafinil (Provigil) and a new sustained release methylphenidate (Ritalin). One of our docs has used Provigil empirically, with some benefit in patients who had side effects with Ritalin. I think there is a lot of variability with the use of these drugs in brain tumor centers. I don't know of anyone with particular expertise to be honest. Chris [Meyers]

Sat Sep 30 2000 7:37 AM

Dear Robert, Re your questions about Mexico: We went to the Hospital San Martin in Tijuana, which is known as the American Metabolic Institute in the U.S. In addition to doing a lot of the holistic kinds of things other clinics down there do, the doctor there has been using an autologous vaccine for about fifteen years. He makes it from the patient's tumor cells if he can get them (I was able to have Stel's paraffin block from her surgery sent to him). If he can't get tumor, he uses blood or urine to get what he needs. Like the vaccines being tried in the U.S., the objective of this vaccine is to teach the white blood cells to fight the tumor. Before we went down there, I spent more than five weeks looking into the treatment, the doctor, the method. I spoke to three other GBM patients or their families who had been to the clinic fourteen years ago, eight years ago, and this year. They all had striking results and are doing very well today even though they were each given a few weeks to a few months to live when they went down there. I also talked to a variety of other patients who had different types of cancer and said they benefited from the treatment. Although I knew there could be a lot of patients out there who had not benefited and wished I could have had specific numbers and results from trials, etc., I was impressed enough from my conversations with most of these people that they were intelligent, not true believers when they went there, capable of making considered judgments, and telling me the truth about their experience to decide that it offered promise to Stel. I had also checked with several researchers in the alternative medicine field who either had a positive view toward the treatment and the doctor or were neutral. I found no negative information.

The hospital itself is very small—seven rooms—but quite pleasant. They've created a little oasis there in the midst of a very busy, clamorous commercial area of Tijuana. They also treat many patients out-patient who stay in hotels. The nursing staff is, on the whole, very professional and caring. The main doctor, Dr. Rubio, has an eclectic approach to treatment—he'll use low-dose radiation, low-dose chemo along with his vaccine and the other holistic approaches, and some things, like color therapy, that most of us more skeptical types view with doubt. The vaccine (he also administers what he calls non-specific vaccines that consist, as well as I could determine, of peptides, lipids and such) is given by shot. It takes twenty-one days to culture it, so in the first three weeks the patient undergoes detoxification and gets other kinds of treatment—including Poly-MVA and the non-specific vaccine shots. Dr. Rubio is very positive and upbeat and truly believes, I think, that every patient can get better. He seems to be quite knowledgeable across a wide range of cancers but, of course, he's not a brain tumor expert. I never could get a firm figure on how many brain tumor patients they've treated over the last 10-15 years, but while we were there I met two of the BT patients I had been in touch with by phone. There are four other doctors there who take their orders from Dr. Rubio. They're staffed 24 hours a day.

As to money, I gave them a $12,000 cashier's check up front, which was meant to cover all the alternative treatments, including the vaccine. Stel's insurance, Blue Cross, had indicated that her policy would cover 70% of the standard stuff—anti-seizure and other meds, CT scans and MRIs (had to get that in San Diego because Tijuana only has one MRI machine), radiation, hospital care, etc. We stayed there seven weeks (they provide a comfortable double bed in the same room with the patient for the caregiver; it's $35 a day for room and board for the extra person; the largely organic meals are very good) and the bill came to about $55,000 (including the $12,000 I had already paid). We left there in mid-June and I've yet to see anything from Blue Cross indicating they've paid yet, but I've never heard another word from the clinic about money. I brought a lot of medications, supplements, home with me—the home follow-up is an important part of the treatment and is a daunting task—and they've sent me stuff since then and have never asked for an additional dime. Ultimately, I think Blue Cross will probably end up paying about half the costs (I assume they'll balk at some things the clinic says were medically necessary and maybe not pay for 70% of everything) and I'll need to come up with another $10,000 or so. If the treatment had worked for Stel as it seems to have worked for others, we would be going back there for booster vaccine shots every three months or so for the next couple of years and that would cost additional money for air fare and the stay there—maybe $2,000-3,000 each time (since we're on the East Coast). Unfortunately, the treatment didn't seem to be as effective for Stel—maybe because of hydrocephalus and/or extensive radiation damage. However, I must say that the tumor has remained stable all this time without conventional treatment (while we've been struggling with the hydrocephalus question and placement of a shunt). Dr. Rubio thinks she would benefit from follow-up shots and is trying to find a way to help her get further treatment without making the trip there, which we just can't do now. I think the doctor is sincere and not in it just to make money. I've also had good dealings with the small AMI staff in San Diego. It's far from a perfect place—you have to keep on top of doctors and nurses (but that's true in the States, too); the language barrier can be a problem; they're not always efficient—but I was impressed with the care and kindness provided. The wife of a man who was there with lung cancer while we were there (he died a few weeks after he went home) told me she was glad they had been at the clinic during those weeks because she felt it was a much more positive experience than they would have had at Kaiser in the States (the doctors there had told her husband from the outset that there was nothing they could do for him). At least they had some good time together. I don't know the outcome for other patients who were there.

I wish I could report the kind of dramatic results other BT patients told me of. It was a very difficult time for me—watching, waiting, hoping to see positive things happening. Stel had a few remarkable days there when we all thought she was taking off, but they didn't last. It was nerve-wracking and heart-wrenching for me—and lonely. Only one friend from L.A. managed to make it down a couple of times. I'm convinced, however, that this clinic isn't a money-grubbing operation just out to fleece gullible, vulnerable patients. Nearly all the patients and caregivers I met there—all from the U.S. or Canada—were intelligent, well-informed people who had, in many cases, tried what their home country had to offer before they came there. Gotta run to the hospital now—Stel is being treated for urinary tract and blood infections. All the best, Kay

Sun Oct 01 2000 9:23 PM

Dear Dr. Torres-Trejo, I have read wonderful comments about your caring efforts to help patients on the Brain Tumor List and so am directing this message to you. [Explanation of Stel's history.] Unfortunately, we are in the Washington, D.C. area at the present time, where I have found it extremely difficult to obtain the comprehensive, specialized treatment for her that I believe might give her some chance to regain some functioning, in addition to treatment for the tumor itself. Since we lived in Los Angeles for many years and have more friends who could be helpful there than here, I'm thinking seriously of trying to get her to L.A. This will undoubtedly be a difficult and costly undertaking, but worth it if she can receive the kind of treatment I am looking for at UCLA.

Because of the unusualness of her condition and its severity, I believe she needs a comprehensive treatment plan, encompassing neuro-oncology, neurosurgery, neurology, and neuro-psychiatry. I am particularly interested in finding doctors who are familiar with research on medications that have helped patients in states of akinetic mutism—.e.g., Ritalin, Parkinson's and Altzheimer's medications—and would be willing to treat Stella with them. At the moment, she is very much alive but has no life. If there is a chance that a medication or other treatment could help her regain some functioning, I want to try it. Doctors here, who are not well versed in the research, are reluctant to try these medications because of fear of seizures or of making things worse. Things could hardly be much worse, and I want to try anything that might help Stella. I am also interested in considering a change in her anti-seizure medication (Tegretol) to a newer one. Can I find the doctors and treatment at UCLA that I'm seeking? Would there be any possibility that she could be evaluated on an in-patient basis? Thanks, Kay Loveland

Mon Oct 02 2000 10:59 PM

Dear Dr. Torres-Trejo, Thank you for your quick response. I would like to have Stella's case presented to the Brain Tumor Board and will try to get all the materials together to send you in the next few days. Kay Loveland

Mon Oct 02 2000 11:02 PM

Dear Stacy, Thanks for your note and phone call. I will call you tomorrow or the next day to discuss how I can manage things so Stella can have an out-patient evaluation at Duke. I will deeply appreciate whatever assistance you can provide. Kay

Wed Oct 04 2000 6:37 AM

Dear Deborah, Unfortunately, there's no sign yet that the shunt has had any positive effect. Stel was at home for three weeks, but a week ago the doctor put her back in the hospital because of urinary tract and blood infections. I thought she'd be coming home tomorrow, but last night her fever spiked up again for the first time in several days and they took blood cultures, so I guess she'll continue to be in the hospital for more antibiotics.

I've been going crazy trying to find a neurologist here who knows about the medications that have helped some people in Stel's condition. Finally, a stroke of luck yesterday—a neurologist who knows more than I do about them, has worked with patients with akinetic mutism, is willing to try different meds with Stel, AND works a block from our apartment and is willing to come to the apartment to see her when she gets home. I all but kissed the guy! Now if she can just come home, we can hope fervently that this bit of luck will continue and she'll respond to something. Love, Kay

Thu Oct 05 2000 9:36 PM

Thanks so much, Stacy, for your message. It's good to know you're there. Hopefully, this lucky break in finding a doctor here will engender more good luck and Stella will respond to some of the medications. It would be the gift of a lifetime to see her smile, to hear her voice again. Kay

Fri Oct 06 2000 2:45 PM

Kay, Steve passed away at 3 a.m. 10/5/00, two years to the day from his original brain tumor surgery. I am hurting so much, in a different way from the grief of losing his essential "Steve-ness" to the radiation damage. Now it's over, and I have to find a way to cope with the complete loss of my dearest love. He went into respiratory distress (rattling from mucus vibrating the vocal cords—he was too weak to cough it up, though I tried everything possible to thin the secretions and help him cough). I hope you and Stel are able to get her the help you are striving for. Love, Phyllis

Fri Oct 06 2000 10:04 PM

Dear Phyllis, I'm so stunned and saddened at this news. This disease just hits you in the solar plexus over and over again. We never know where the next blow is going to come from—out of left field; from a totally different direction than anticipated. That's what I fear—I'm going along on one or two tracks thinking if I can just get the right treatments things may be okay, but who knows what terrible surprise could come along to make all that meaningless—respiratory failure, infection, god knows what. I'm so deeply sorry. I can feel how much you're hurting. I guess all we can do is be grateful for the years we had together and the memories of the loving times we shared. It's so hard when we expected so many more. My kindest thoughts are with you. Kay

Tue Oct 10 2000 6:36 AM

Dear Jeanne, It's good to hear from you. We're going through hell here. Thanks for the name of the neurologist. I will contact him. I just had a stroke of good luck last week when I found a neurologist here who has worked with people in Stel's condition using Provigil, Parkinson's meds, etc., and his office is a block from our apartment and he's coming to the apartment late this afternoon. I pray that Stel will respond to something. I'll be in touch. Kay

Wed Oct 11 2000 6:13 AM

Jeanne, I'd really appreciate it if you could send me everything listed on your protocol—plus the multi-vitamin and bromelain I already ordered—because I just don't have the time to be running around trying to assemble them. This would take a large load off my shoulders. Whatever you can send right away, please do. Then send the special order stuff when you get it.

The neurologist was supposed to have come yesterday evening but didn't show up, which upset me. Got to call his office first thing this morning to see what happened and implore him to get over here ASAP. It's taken too long to find someone who can prescribe these meds as it is. How I wish we still lived in L.A. or the Bay Area, near a major BT center. The DC area is a no-man's land when it comes to this. NIH sits there but is basically useless to a patient who can't qualify for a clinical trial—they're even studying radiation damage there, but Stel's too non-functional to be eligible. Hopkins is impossible—even the oncologist can't get a call back from anyone there, and they're so conservative in their approach anyway.

I'd like to call you today or tomorrow to talk about the patients you've dealt with who have radiation damage. Do you know of anyone who has tried hyperbaric oxygen? Thanks for this help. Kay

Thu Oct 12 1000 5:06 AM

Dear Rita, I haven't written before, but I've followed Margaret's odyssey through your messages. I'm so deeply sorry for all she—and you—have gone through. My partner Stel and I continue on with the battles, still hoping, despite great odds, ultimately to win the war. But the obstacles seem to grow by the day. Please know you have my deepest sympathy. Kay Loveland

Thu Oct 12 2000 10:18 PM

Pat, Thanks for your message. Unfortunately, Stel isn't doing any better. In fact, she's sleeping almost all the time. The shunt has had no effect so far, unless it's made things worse. I had a lucky break this week, though, when I found a neurologist near our apartment who knows about the medications I've wanted to try and is willing to work with us. I was so desperate before I found him that I was planning to take her down to Duke in an ambulance for out-patient evaluation. But I feel pretty comfortable with this doctor and that he will try the things that might be helpful. He said he didn't think Ritalin is likely to work and wanted to start with Provigil, which he says is a neat drug that doesn't have too many side effects and wakes a lot of narcoleptics up. We started today with half a pill and will work up to two pills over the next several days. There was no response today. I pray as we go up it will have an effect, but I'm afraid to hope. I've been through this watching and waiting so much, and the roller coaster ride of hoping and then having my hopes dashed to the ground. But if it doesn't work by next week, we'll move on to the Parkinson's meds.

I've been in touch with UCLA and their BT Board is looking at everything this week and will give me their recommendations. I'm still thinking I may want to try to get her out there so we'll be closer to some old friends who could be helpful. It would be a gigantic undertaking, though. Thanks for asking about Stel. Hope you're doing okay. Kay

Sun Oct 15 2000 6:14 AM

Dear Phyllis, Your message to the List is beautiful. Know that I am with you in your pain and grieving, as I watch and wait here to see whether the new meds "bring Stella back" at all. All of this is so painful and so overwhelmingly difficult, and it's made even more so by knowing that I can't have any communication with the partner I've shared everything with for so long. Your message helps me prepare for what I hope won't come but must, nevertheless, steel myself for. May the days become less painful and your memories of Steve in good times together sustain you. Love, Kay

Mon Oct 16 2000 4:20 AM

Dear Michael, Unfortunately I've learned more than I ever wanted to know about the detrimental effects of radiotherapy in the past several months. It's not something much talked about by doctors and I wasn't at all prepared for what has happened to my partner Stel. But your father is in the early days of treatment and, hopefully, won't experience the delayed effects that Stel apparently is suffering from. There are stages of radiation effects. The early ones, while therapy is going on and in the weeks immediately following, usually resolve themselves with no serious after effects, I understand. Stel came through the initial period with no severe problems. Then there can be early delayed and late delayed effects, happening from months to years after treatment. Early delayed, again, probably will resolve itself. Late delayed, they say, is permanent, often progressive, and there's not a lot that can be done to treat it. For the past nine months, Stel has progressively lost functioning to the point that she now can do nothing for herself and is mute. Throughout most of that time, I was frantically trying to find out from doctors why she wasn't doing better since the tumor was (and remains) stable. Only in the last 3-4 months did I find out about late-delayed radiation effects (she had radiation in the summer of 1999 and a stereotactic radiosurgery boost in December 1999), which some doctors believe is the primary cause of all of her deficits. Other doctors think she's suffering from the accumulation of all the traumas inflicted on her poor brain—surgery, radiation, chemo, the tumor itself. Among the few treatments that sometimes help people with radiation damage are a variety of medications including Provigil and various Parkinson's drugs. I've just started Stel on this road, hoping she'll respond to something. If she doesn't, there isn't much in the way of other options.

I'm sure this is more than you wanted to know about this subject now. And, as I say, your dad is at an early point and may well not experience the kind of problems Stel has—I certainly hope he doesn't. But I think it's important that we know more about what can happen as a result of the treatments themselves. We're so busy fighting the tumor and if we're lucky enough to get that under control, think things should get better. It's devastating to find out that the treatment may cause as many or more problems than the tumor and may, ultimately, be the cause of the person's death. (See the recent message from Phyllis Walker.) I hope for the best for your dad and you. Kay

Mon Oct 16 2000 3:52 PM

Vanessa, The terrible struggle continues here. Stel came through shunt surgery in late August fine, but so far there's been no indication of any positive benefit. It could still happen, but as weeks pass, I think it's less and less likely. She's been on antibiotics for a couple of infections over the past month—damned urinary tract infection from catheter. Strange to me that in seven weeks in Mexico she never got an infection because they gave her what they called an antiseptic, but here they don't know anything about that, and within 2-3 weeks of having a catheter in, she got an infection, as she did last year after her surgery.

I'm now working with a neurologist whose office is a block away to give Stel some of the medications that might help her. He started her on one med last week and we'll know in a couple of days if it's having any effect—so far, nothing. If not, he'll move on to Parkinson's drugs. For me, it's more watching, waiting, hoping, fearing—purgatory if ever there was. Stel mostly sleeps now, and when she can manage to wake up a bit, she's usually staring off in space. Once in a while I can engage her in eye contact and feel she is registering what I'm saying to her. I can't tell you how lonely it is. I've bought a bunch of CDs of some of the great old songs—Cole Porter, Gershwin—that I know she knows by heart from her days of singing them in a chorus in high school and I sing along with them to her. At times she's clearly been paying attention. Whatever else, it's a solace to me—so many of them are wonderfully romantic and express so much of what I feel for her.

So far as we know, the tumor is still stable, at least as of September 11th. She'll have another MRI next week and we'll see. The $64,000 question is what to do next for treatment for it. If we could be fortunate enough to get it to start shrinking, it might help her, but adding more toxins to the brain tissue is very worrisome. There's no real consensus about what's causing her problems—radiation damage or mixture of treatments and tumor. (Actually, the Brain Tumor Board at UCLA will review her case this week and let me know what they would recommend in terms of treatment at this point.)

I've told Stel I think she's gone into hibernation until all this shit resolves itself. In fact, I do have a sense that after the many trials and tribulations she's endured in her life, this was just too much, and she checked out. But who knows? One thinks that after thirty-one years of so deep and close a relationship, there will always be some form of communication there and you'll know instinctively what the other is feeling, but now I know that's all just romantic notions. Confronting the sphinx that Stel has become, I don't really have any more of a clue than anyone else. I just love her with all my heart and soul and keep repeating that to her, hoping that somehow, somewhere in the deep recesses of her poor battered brain, it registers and makes a difference. Despite the track record, I'm keeping the faith here, still believing it's possible for Stella to re-emerge from her stupor, smile her wonderful smile, chuckle her infectious laugh, and say in her melodious voice, "Hi, Kate, I'm back." Stay in touch. Love, Kay

Wed Oct 18 2000 9:28 PM

Dear Heather, I'm excited, and perplexed, to receive your message—excited that you're going to try hyperbaric oxygen for your mother and perplexed as to why Henry Friedman didn't mention it to me as an option for Stel when I corresponded with him last month. I've been interested in HBOT for several months but haven't found much mainstream support for it in regard to brain tumors, so I'm very happy to know that Friedman thinks it's a viable treatment for radiation damage. Please let me know how it goes, and how your mother responds. I'm very anxious to know about this.

I'm also excited to know that your mother has come out of her apathy and is laughing, joking and feeding herself. Do you have any idea how this happened? Is it a result of changing the anti-seizure medication? I've seen mention of others who have improved when they changed seizure medications, and I really want to try that for Stel. What else could have caused her to get better? Any ideas?

I'm glad you ignored the neuro-psychologist's suggestion of the hospice route. I think doctors are too quick to start pushing that. I hope so much that HBOT works for your mother. PLEASE keep me posted!! Kay

Wed Oct 18 2000 9:51 PM

Jeanne, I got the supplements. I'm hoping so much that they, along with the meds, will have a positive effect on Stel. We've just got to get her functioning to some extent again. The UCLA BT Board looked at her scans, etc. today and told me they think her latest MRI, from five weeks ago, looks a little better than previous ones. That's the first I've heard that. Here, they just say it looks the same. I can't see much difference myself, but I hope the more practiced eyes at UCLA have got it right. She'll have another MRI next week, and how I'd love to see more visible positive change. Keep your fingers crossed! Thanks so much for the phone call the other day. It helped a lot. Kay

Wed Oct 18 2000 10:15 PM

Dear Dr. Friedman, I just received a message from Heather Wilson about her mother's problems apparently due to radiation damage. She said you had told her hyperbaric oxygen therapy is a proven treatment for tissue that has been damaged by radiation, and she is planning to find such treatment for her mother. I've been interested in hyperbaric oxygen treatment for Stel and am wondering why you didn't mention it as a possibility for her when we corresponded last month. I'd appreciate your thoughts. Thanks, Kay Loveland

Wed Oct 18 2000 10:54 PM

To BT List: With permission, I'm forwarding this message from Phyllis Walker to all of you because of the importance of the subject matter. She and I have had a very rude awakening in the past several months about the serious consequences that radiation therapy can have on brain tumor patients. Even if you're fortunate enough to get the tumor under control, you may find yourself struggling to deal with the deleterious effects of the treatments that contained the tumor. The following is Phyllis' message:

"Reading your message to Michael was a sad reminder for me of everything that happened to Steve. But it was very well expressed and any BT patient and caregiver needs to know about these possibilities. I still don't know whether it was the whole brain radiation (WBR). Gamma Knife propagandists would have us believe that WBR is the real culprit, but who knows? Not long ago I received a newsletter called 'Another Perspective,' [the publication for the International Radiosurgery Support Assn.]. The entire issue was devoted to metastatic brain tumors (and the benefits of treatment with Gamma Knife for this condition). This is a quote:

'Significant neurotoxicity has been reported with the use of WBRT. Acute effects include hair loss (alopecia), nausea, vomiting, lethargy, otitis media and severe cerebral edema. Though some of these effects can be transient, dermatitis, alopecia, and otitis media can persist for months after irradiation. Chronic effects are even more serious, and these include atrophy, leukoencephalopathy, radiation necrosis, neurological deterioration and dementia. Reports of development of severe radiation induced dementia have varied between 11% in one-year survivors to 50% in those surviving two years.'

"NOW THEY TELL ME THIS!!!! I swear to you that none of the medical people (radio/oncologists for either WBR or GK, the oncologist or the neurosurgeon) even hinted at these possibilities (except for hair loss and some fatigue for a while). I read all the radiation pamphlets at the Radiation Center, and none of them mentioned any side-effects except short-term. Here's another quote (this one from my journal entry prior to Steve's Jan 2000 GK treatment): 'Steve will not lose his hair this time, should feel nothing during the 45 min. of radiation, and will probably not have any side effects. (There's a SLIM chance he may have some temporary weakness on the left side, if there's any radiation 'bouncing off' the targeted area. This is why the preferred treatment is radiation—because the tumor's location is close to a part of the brain that controls motor function. So traditional surgery might definitely result in some weakness, whereas radiation might not') This is only GK I was talking about here. And surgery WAS his first treatment in 1997, for a solitary right temporal lobe tumor about the size of an egg, which seemed to be "in situ," not spidery. Ten rounds of WBR followed. The GK treatment I wrote about above was for recurrences of two grape-sized nodules.

"You can share this with the List unless you think it is too negative. It might prompt someone to push for more information from their docs, and maybe one kind of radiation would be preferable over another. I think that I read somewhere that part of what's going on is that BT patients never had much of a prognosis in the past and probably died before the long-term side effects surfaced. Now the survival time is a little longer, so…we get these nasty surprises. But…as I recently told someone, Steve and I would probably have gone along with ALL the treatment recommendations because the alternative might be that he would not have had eighteen good months that he did have from the time of the BT diagnosis. What else can you do but try everything and trust that the doctors 'know best.' At least I USED to think that before this last four months became the worst nightmare I've ever lived through. Now I know that a lot of the brain is still a mystery to the medical people. I used to get SOOO frustrated because none of them could explain REALLY what was happening with Steve. They just did a lot of guessing, mostly, and didn't always try to BS me that they had a handle on his condition. As with all of us on the List, I became a pest to the ns and onc, and sometimes took it upon myself to do for Steve what I thought was best (like readjusting the Decadron taper). I have learned SO much from reading the List postings, as well as the Merck Manual, plus invaluable information from the American Brain Tumor Association.

"I hope this doesn't sound too bitter and cynical. When all is said and done, 'Ya gotta do what ya gotta do.' Hope all is as well as it can be for you, under the circumstances. You are doing everything you possibly can for Stel, and on some level I believe she knows it, and Steve knew that I was totally 'there' for him as well, despite my occasional lapses of patience and fits of temporary depression. They know. But that doesn't take away the pain of not being able to communicate with the most important person in our lives. Love, Phyllis"

Wed Oct 18 2000 11:38 PM

Dear Phyllis, Good to hear from you. Stel just tried her first new med this week, and it didn't work. I'm seeing the doctor tomorrow to decide on the next one to try. I'm praying one of them will work for her, but the watching, waiting, and worrying is crazy-making. I agree with you that BT caregivers and patients need to have more forewarning about these possibilities when they go into treatment. It's a terrible subject to have to bring up, but it's just not fair to gloss over it and leave us completely at sea when we start seeing manifestations of these problems. It is, as you said, a nasty surprise. Like you, we got no information at the time Stel was going through radiation that alerted us to the serious consequences to come. I think they may have mentioned in passing that there could be long-term somnolence syndrome, but who in the hell knows what that means? Regarding WBRT, I have seen mention in medical journals that radiation damage is more likely to result from whole brain radiation. Stel didn't have whole brain—it was called something else and utilized fields that took in a lot but didn't encompass everything.

I'm sure Stel is suffering from its effects. I know, though, that the stereotactic radiosurgery increased the problems. She never functioned as well in any way—and particularly cognitively—from the time she had the procedure. I wrote the doctor who did it about what she was experiencing and he didn't respond until I went to the director of CINN. Finally, I talked to him on the phone and he said he doubted very much that the radiosurgery caused her difficulties. He thought it was metabolic, but there's never been any indication of that. I have no doubt Stel is worse off because of the procedure; but it's a double-edged sword because the procedure also stopped the tumor in its tracks. If fortune had smiled on Stel, she could have had some very decent months since January. Instead, it's just been hell. What struck me about the lack of follow-up after the radiosurgery is that it's no wonder the doctors tell us there are minimal risks; if they don't follow up and don't know what happens to patients, then they can't tell anyone about those who don't fare so well.

It's true that doctors and scientists really know very little about the brain and even less about adult brain regeneration. It's all new territory. And so those of us having to deal with the horror of brain tumors find ourselves wandering in the wilderness with no guide. We have to make these terrible decisions for which there are no good alternatives. And we have to live with them. I wouldn't wish this nightmare on my worst enemy.

I hope, as you say, that on some level Stel knows how much I care and how hard I'm trying to help her. Having been hit with the mack truck of a BT, I've found out there isn't any special communication with my beloved. Stel is as much an enigma to me as to everyone else these days—something I could never have imagined in my wildest dreams. She was always one to express all of her feelings to me, a passionate, opinionated, lively being and now she lies mute and inert in bed, her face a blank slate except when it records some displeasure. It's just so unbelievable. My adored Stella reduced to this, and in so short a time.

I hope you're doing okay. Let me know if you find good ways of dealing with your anger and grief. Love, Kay

Wed Oct 18 2000 11:53 PM

[From Dr. Friedman]: Two reasons [why I didn't recommend HBOT for Stella]—the risk of using hyperbaric 02 in someone in whom you suspect active tumor may be present—a real concern for Stel. The other is that you must be able to be somewhat independent to go into a hyperbaric chamber and comply with instructions. We do not do it for someone who cannot function in this fashion. Henry

Thu Oct 19 2000 6:18 AM

Dr. Torres-Trejo, I greatly appreciated your willingness to talk at length last night. I realized afterwards that there were some questions I had about the PET scan that perhaps you could answer for me. You indicated that PET scans are tricky. What is the likelihood that a reading of viable tumor on a PET scan may be wrong? Would radiation damage (as opposed to necrosis) look the same as tumor on the PET scan? I wondered whether on Stella's scan you could tell whether there is radiation necrosis in other areas of the brain not adjacent to the tumor? I'm thinking of the diffuse white matter changes shown throughout her brain on her MRIs and whether, if any of that represents necrosis, you would be able to see that on the PET scan. If you have a moment to reply about these issues, I'd appreciate it. Many thanks, Kay

Thu Oct 19 2000 6:28 AM

Dr. F: What is the risk of HBOT if you suspect active tumor? Kay

Thu Oct 19 2000 7:33 AM

Dear Peter, Stel's case was presented to the Brain Tumor Board at UCLA yesterday and I talked to a very nice doctor about their thoughts last night. He actually said they thought the tumor looked a little smaller on the September MRI, which is the first time I've heard that. I pray they're right and that we'll see something encouraging on her scan next week. The heartbreaking part, though, is even if we do, she will probably still be in her helpless state. The first medication we tried hasn't done anything positive for her. I'm going to see the neurologist this morning (since I can't stand to sit around waiting for phone calls, as I did yesterday) to discuss which med we'll try next. I'm so scared we'll run through everything and have no change. The UCLA doctor suggested another medication that I'd read a little about that I'm going to mention to the neurologist. Also, he recommended a mild chemo drug [Accutane] that I had already told the oncologist I'd be interested in trying against the tumor, so that bolstered my feeling that that's what we should try next. I'll let you know how things go. Kay

Fri Oct 20 2000 7:59 AM

[From Dr. Friedman]: Tumor can aggressively start to grow under the high oxygen levels. Henry

Sun Oct 22 2000 6:29 AM

Dear Steve, Just wondered if you still think you could perform courier duty in 2-3 weeks? I'm still vacillating, but leaning more in the direction of trying to get the vaccine here. Unfortunately, there's nothing new to report. Stel sleeps almost all the time. The first med didn't do anything. She's now on a Parkinson's drug for the last couple of days, but there's been no change. It's a tiny dose, though, and I think anything that might work is going to have to be at higher levels. Thanks, Kay

Tue Oct 24 2000 9:32 AM

[To BT List]: My husband and I went back to see his surgeon yesterday to have his staples removed. After a brief conversation with him, I mentioned that I have met on line a handful of GBM survivors that have been thriving for years. He told me that their pathology reports were probably wrong and that they do not have GBMs. So with that in mind, I thought all of you GBM survivors would like to know that our brilliant surgeon just downgraded all of your tumors! Thankfully, we don't have to deal with him anymore. Julia

Tue Oct 24 2000 9:15 PM

Julia, My partner Stel's surgeon made a similar comment as she dispensed her usual quotient of doom and gloom—along the lines of "we don't know what their diagnosis was." I replied that the people on this List seem quite capable of reporting back what their doctors and MRI and pathology reports say and, given that, I've encountered more survivors who have beat the median by a long shot than I ever would have expected in light of the miserable statistics that are always quoted. I surmise that if the statistics were entirely correct, I could count on two hands, at most, the number of long-term survivors I would have encountered in the last year and a half. There are at least double or triple that number that I've heard of. Stel can be included among those who have certainly beat the median by a distance (eighteen months and counting), but sadly eleven months of that time has been mostly ghastly. Fortunately, others have had better luck. Still hoping for brighter days, Kay

Wed Oct 25 2000 6:25 AM

Dear Bob, I just saw your message of 9/15. Thanks so much for your kindness in writing me directly and your caring words for Stel and me. I'm writing you one day after an MRI that, for the first time in ten months, shows tumor growth. Stel's surgeon, whose forte is not looking on the hopeful side, said she thinks the tumor has grown so large that it's blocking out the ventricles on the scan. Maybe so, but it seems to me if there were that much change in six weeks' time I would be seeing a significant worsening of Stel's condition, which I haven't. It's bad enough as it is, but it hasn't gotten much worse. At any rate, I measured the tumor, as I have all the ones since last November, and it does appear to be about

1/8th of an inch bigger at its widest and longest points. This is not good news, but it's also not extremely rapid growth. I'm scared this morning, though, and worrying about what to do next and whether I can get the doctors here to do more—and worried, of course, about whether any further treatment will help.

Stel has been on Poly-MVA since we went to Mexico in May. In the past two months, I've been giving her five teaspoons a day. For the past month, she's been entirely off of Decadron, so I believed this would provide the optimum opportunity for the Poly to work if it was going to. It doesn't seem to have done anything, given the MRI. And I've seen no clinical improvement in Stel during this time that would have made me think it was working. So, it appears another treatment that has worked for some isn't working for Stel. As for the AMI vaccine, that, too, seems to have failed. If only the Poly and vaccine could have done for Stel what they've apparently done for Martha Baker. How my heart aches that Stel couldn't have such good fortune, but I regret to say that has been the story of her life in many ways.

I'm going to ask the oncologist to start Stel on Accutane and Temodar. I hate the thought of it, but I don't see any other avenue now. I hope she will agree. Henry Friedman had declined to give Stel any more treatment because of her current status (not talking, not moving); he felt it might make things worse. I went along with that, but wish I hadn't now and had started her a month or two ago. Things really couldn't get much worse, and there is always the possibility that they could get better if the tumor could shrink some. Also, there's a lot of swelling now, so I guess we'll have to put her back on the Decadron for that. If Stel can improve, then maybe I can get her back on the medication regimen (stimulants, Parkinson's meds, etc.) we started in the last two weeks to try to make her more alert and functional. So far nothing positive had happened with that, but it's still early in the process, which I wish I could have started six months ago, or at least three months ago, but it took me until three weeks ago to find a neurologist here who knew enough about the meds to administer them to someone in Stel's situation.

The odds are very long and lengthening this morning, but I'm going to continue fighting for Stel's valuable life, despite constantly being pushed toward hospice because "it would be easier on me." This is Stel's LIFE we're talking about, which is in far more danger than mine right now. In my view, our lives are of equal value and therefore I'll devote my energies to the one most at risk at the moment.

I'm so glad Poly has helped Roberta. I hope things are still going well with you. I'm deeply appreciative of your support and concern. All the best, Kay

Wed Oct 25 2000 6:47 AM

Jeanne, Thought I'd forward to you this message that I just wrote because it has the very latest information—not good. I hate to put Stel back on Decadron, but it seems we're going to have to. I've been giving her the bromelain several times a day, but it hasn't seemed to help with the swelling. Several months ago I was trying both the bromelain and boswellin at the same time, but they never seemed to have an effect on Stel. Unfortunately, nothing seems to have an effect, except perhaps the radiation, which helped to put her in the state she's in now. If you have any further thoughts about things to do, please call me today if you can. I'd appreciate hearing from you. Thanks, Kay

Wed Oct 25 2000 10:20 PM

[To BT List]: As promised, I wanted to let you know about mom's initial evaluation with one of the doctors at the hyperbaric medicine center at Hospital University of Pennsylvania. After a rundown of the side effects, which include decreased lung capacities and an increase in nearsightedness (which return to baseline once treatment has ended), he (Dr. James Clark) told us that he has had lots of success with radiation damage to the head and neck areas. Not as much success with brain damage. BUT he wants to get mom in as soon as possible. He's moved her to the top of the waiting list. The treatments last for over two hours. They usually do thirty treatments which are done daily (Mon-Sat) for five weeks.

Today mom had an MRI. It once again showed that the tumor is stable. The radiologist showed us where the brain damage is. It's pretty diffuse. The radiologist was absolutely amazed at mom's turnaround. She's pretty confident it was the increase in Ritalin to 15 mg twice a day. We also got her off Depakote and on to Neurontin (which I think has helped. Mom had AWFUL tremors while she was on Depakote) and we started her on a few herbal supplements. It could be a combination of all three. Who knows! We all are just so happy to see the improvement! Once she gets started on the HBOT, I will definitely let you know how it's going. Heather

Thu Oct 26 2000 5:44 AM

Dear Heather, Thanks for the update. It sounds very hopeful for your mom and I'm so happy she's going to get the HBOT. I'm wondering whether the hyperbaric doctor said anything about the effect of HBOT on the tumor itself. It's so wonderful that your mom has turned around with the Ritalin and other things. Unfortunately, Stel had no response to 30 mg of Ritalin twice a day back in July when we tried it. Unfortunately, too, her MRI this week shows some tumor growth for the first time in ten months. It doesn't appear to be a large amount, but I'm very worried and want to get Stel back on chemo treatment for it immediately. I'm seeing the neurologist this morning to see what he says about how this will affect his treatment for alertness and functionality. Given this turn of events, I guess I won't be pushing for HBOT for Stel soon, but I'll be very interested to know how it's going for your mother. I hope her good luck continues. All the best, Kay

Fri Oct 27 2000 6:35 AM

Steve, I don't think I'm going to pursue the vaccine any further; I just don't have enough evidence of its effectiveness. Stel's MRI this week reinforces that conclusion. Of course, as with everything else in the course of this horrid disease, it's unclear as to what is going on. Her surgeon looked at the scan on Tuesday and, in her usual doom and gloom fashion, told me that the tumor had grown and, she thought, now was so big that it was obscuring the view of the ventricles, which apparently have gotten substantially smaller since the shunt was placed (one of the things I had hoped would result from the shunt, but it seems to have had no effect on Stel). She had no encouraging words at all and really discouraged me from pursuing further treatment. Naturally, I was in a state when we came home.

After I looked at the scans, I felt she was painting too black a picture. My unscientific measurements indicated that the tumor might be less than half a centimeter bigger in width and length, not much given the ferocity of how these tumors usually grow. I also just didn't think the tumor could be big enough to obscure the ventricles. If that were the case, it seemed to me I'd be seeing different things happening with Stel. At any rate, I showed the scan to the neurologist yesterday. What a difference a less pessimistic doctor makes. He said he wasn't sure the tumor was any larger because MRI cuts are never exactly the same and unless there's really a substantial increase, it's hard to tell. Also, he thought the ventricles weren't very visible because, again, of a different cut. He said that Stel's surgeon always sees the glass half empty, which I'm well aware of.

At any rate, since it's unclear whether there is new growth, I do want to start her on treatment and am talking to the oncologist about the milder chemo possibilities. I was still juggling the vaccine idea around and had found out how long it could last on ice before use (48 hours) and had talked to AMI about logistics when I found out last night that the woman who did so well with the treatment back in January-February and who, I last heard in August, was coming along very well, died in late September. The tumor grew back, apparently, after she had surgery for a hairline fracture. I understand her recovery was very difficult and she sort of gave up and didn't want any more BT treatment. Her husband thinks, I'm told, that her death didn't result from failure of the vaccine treatment but from her impaired immune system as a result of the chemo she had last year. Who knows. At least she had five or six months of fairly decent life with her family that she probably wouldn't have had if her husband hadn't taken her out of the hospice last January. I remember seeing her laughing when they returned from a trip to the beach back in May when we were in Mexico, and hoping I'd see Stel that way soon. At any rate, I don't think the vaccine is an avenue to pursue further for Stel now.

The UCLA Brain Tumor Board did review Stel's case and the nice doctor there indicated that they really don't know much about Parkinson's meds, etc. They do work with Ritalin and the other stimulant we just tried with Stel that didn't have an effect. I was surprised they aren't doing more. As to treatment for the tumor, he recommended a "mild" chemo that I'm interested in, but the oncologist here is balking because she hasn't used it. I've got to have more discussion with her about it. The doctor at UCLA wanted to see the scan done this week but is out of town until November 13th. It will be interesting to see what he makes of it.

The Parkinson's med we tried for three days last week (tiny dose) didn't do anything for Stel, but I wouldn't expect that it could at such a low level. We then switched to a more powerful stimulant [Adderall] and it has seemed to have an effect in waking her up some. She's been unable to keep her eyes open for several weeks; with this med, she doesn't have that problem and has been awake more. The problem is it seemed to increase her blood pressure. But the doctor said to lower the dose a bit and keep trying it this week and checking her pressure. The pressure can stabilize, he said. If we can use this to wake her up, then he can add in other meds to see whether we can increase her responsiveness. Of course, this will have to be coordinated with any chemo she's on. Also, unfortunately, I had to put her back on the steroid, which she's been free of for almost five weeks, yesterday because of significant swelling shown on the MRI. The neurologist has other ideas of how to deal with this, but the oncologist wouldn't go along. So I'm going to give her the steroid this week and when I see him next week see whether he will take over this aspect of things, too. That's everything for now. Kay

NOTE: Regarding the Mexican vaccine treatment, I'm still not sure what I think about its effectiveness for other patients. I know from what her husband said that Martha Baker had a miraculous resurrection from impending death while she was at the clinic and when I saw her in there in May, she was talking, laughing, and moving her body. I suppose that could have been just a fluke. However, other patients I spoke to on the phone or met at the clinic—Bill Blakley in particular—spoke of coming there after they had received death sentences from mainstream doctors and recovering substantially or completely from their illnesses. In many cases, they were alive years after their treatment at the clinic. None of them seemed to be true believers when they went there; they had sought out alternative treatment when doctors at home had given up on them. On the other hand, to the extent that I have knowledge, I'm not aware of any cancer patients who were at the clinic during the time we were there who are still alive. But patients came and went during that time and I didn't meet all of them, so I can't speak definitively about this. I did learn recently that in the summer of 2001, the clinic was shut down by the Mexican authorities in what the San Diego newspaper called a "months-long crackdown...against alternative health clinics that are operating illegally along the border." According to the article, in the course of the crackdown, the Mexican health department had closed half a dozen clinics that "did not have permits or research protocols to provide experimental treatments." Some were allowed to reopen to offer only conventional care. With reference particularly to AMI, the article stated that the clinic had been raided after it "allegedly twice defied an order to stop treating patients" and had moved its operations to a Tijuana hotel. The article quoted authorities as saying that the clinic offered unproven treatments "including injections made from chicken liver extracts and guinea pig tissue" to patients. (This may have been what Dr. Rubio called "nonspecific vaccine" shots. I was told guinea pigs were used in vaccine production.) They threatened AMI with permanent closure, but a check of its website recently indicates it is still operating almost two years later. Whatever the truth of the matter, I don't believe that Dr. Rubio is a quack who is just in it for the money. I think he sincerely believes he can and does help people. I never felt pressured by

AMI to pay anything beyond the $12,000 I paid up front and my $35 a day room and board, which was certainly reasonable. It took months for Blue Cross finally to make payment and it tried to get out of it at first by claiming that Stel's policy only covered emergency treatment in a foreign country. But after I appealed and cited three instances in which Blue Cross representatives had assured me and AMI that it would pay 70% of necessary medical expenses, it reversed its decision and actually ended up paying the whole bill above the $12,000 I had already paid. AMI waited patiently throughout the whole process and indicated to me when Blue Cross was balking that if the appeal failed, it would work with me to come to a reasonable accommodation on the bill.

Sat Oct 28 2000 7:02 AM

Dear Phyllis, Stel is about the same, and I am coping about the same, although the thought of dark winter nights, cold weather, and the holidays coming up makes me wonder how I'll get through the coming weeks. I'm pushing friends to pencil me in as one of their "meetings" so that I know I have regular visits coming. That gives me a psychological boost. A couple of friends are doing well at this so far. The neurologist is trying different meds. The first couple didn't do anything—although the dose of the second one was very low and it might be effective at higher doses, which can be tried later. The third med, a stimulant, has seemed to have some effect in waking her up. She's been awake for hours at a time—at least her eyes have been open. It hasn't made her any more responsive, but first we have to wake her up. Unfortunately, the drug also increased her blood pressure substantially. We've cut back the dose to experiment with it this week to see if the pressure stabilizes. Hopefully it will.

The latest MRI caused some concerns. Her surgeon and the neurologist disagree as to whether the tumor is bigger. The ventricles are definitely smaller—what I wanted to achieve with the shunt, but there's been no corresponding improvement on Stel's part—more frustration. So it's unclear whether there's any new growth, but I want to get some treatment going for Stel. I've been talking to the oncologist about some of the "milder" chemos—Accutane, Temodar, Tamoxifen. She wanted to talk to Friedman again. I don't want to put Stel on a rough chemo but would like to try to do something to see if we can get this beast to stop growing, if it is, and to shrink it a little, if at all possible. Hopefully, I'll get this resolved this week. More horrible decisions to make.

You said you're not fighting your grief, just "going with the flow (of tears) every day." I think this is the best thing you can do. As you said in one of your messages, you just have to go through the pain. There's no way to skip over it. Of course, I'm already grieving, as you were, at the many losses so far and at seeing Stel in such sad circumstances. As to your worry that in some way you failed Steve, you're not alone in these thoughts. Given the enormity of what we're dealing with and the complete uncertainty in the medical world as to what works and what doesn't, I don't think there's any way any of us can keep from having these nagging worries. And, of course, you never know what might have happened if you'd taken a different fork in the road. Usually, that doesn't matter so much because it's not a life or death matter. In these decisions, it could be, and you don't know which road could lead to life. I worry now that if I hadn't known about the stereotactic radiosurgery in Chicago, Stel wouldn't have done that and wouldn't have immediately had such deficits that have grown greater with each passing month. She would have gone on a chemo and maybe it would have worked and she would still be functioning halfway decently (but the sneaky bastard, late radiation damage might have kicked in and caused her the same problems even without the radiosurgery). But who knows? I know the radiosurgery stopped the tumor from growing. There's no certainty that the chemo would have and if it hadn't, then I guess she would have soon had the same deficits from the growing tumor that she seems to have had from the radiosurgery, and she probably wouldn't still be here at all. Whether that's a blessing is another profound question. It is for me in the sense that I can still hug and kiss her and tell her I love her, but it's not in all other ways for her or me. Nevertheless, I still think where there's life there may be hope of improvement and that keeps me going for the moment.

Believe me, it's not upsetting to hear from you. Please stay in touch; I appreciate your friendship. I hope as the weeks go by, you'll begin to feel less intense pain. Stel and I will keep on keeping on here for the time being. Love, Kay

Sun Oct 29 2000 11:01 PM

Jeanne, Just wanted to let you know that Stel's neurologist didn't share the gloomy view of her surgeon about the MRI. He's not even sure the tumor has grown because he says the cut was different from the previous scan. His view was much more in line with my own after I looked more closely at the scan. So, I don't know whether we're dealing with growth or not. The oncologist is talking to Friedman about a new chemo. I have my doubts he'll suggest anything because he's not wanted to do anything in the last couple of months. I told the oncologist if that's still his view, I want to go ahead anyway. I'm debating Temodar, Tamoxifen, Accutane. She seems reluctant on the Accutane and I have to talk to her further about that. Oh god, I hate all of this, and all of the uncertainty of not knowing whether something will work or not.

In the meantime, the neurologist has Stel on a stimulant, Adderall, which has seemed to have some effect in waking her up. But it also affected her blood pressure and we're playing around with the dosage. So far, so good. Of course, if she goes on a chemo that makes her sleepy, as Temodar did, that will work against these efforts. What to do, what to do?? She's doing pretty well vis a vis the infections she had, seems to be over them. Temperature is back to normal. She's back on Decadron this week, but I want to talk to the neurologist when I see him about his suggestion of putting her on Lasix with a potassium supplement instead. The oncologist didn't want to do that, but seems to me it can't cause worse problems than the steroid. That's the story for now. Better get to bed. Kay

Mon Oct 30 2000 6:53 AM

Dear Jeanne, I have a few questions and comments about some things in your welcome message: <As for Decadron v. Lasix for swelling, the Lasix will only reduce fluid volume, but not interfere with inflammatory prostaglandins.> I don't understand the significance of this. If you can reduce the fluid with Lasix, what real benefit are you losing by not affecting the prostaglandins? <Also, the Decadron has the benefit of being stimulating/arousing and you would lose that if you switch to the Lasix.> I've never been able to see any significant effects of Decadron with Stel, no matter how high or low the dose. <If you do decide for the Lasix, it will deplete B vitamins (which are essential for brain function and repair) so you might want to ensure Stel gets her multi (or a B complex) together with the Lasix.> Would she be getting enough B complex with the multi you sent her? I'm giving that to her.

As for how I'm doing, I'm barely hanging in there this morning. In fact, I'm feeling really bad. Usually I feel somewhat up in the morning, looking to a new day when something positive might happen. But the day after day of sameness, coupled with the need to make medication/chemo decisions, is getting to me today. Also thinking of winter approaching and long, dark nights, and how I'll get through the holiday season, whether friends here will really make an effort to help me through that or just get so wrapped up in their own shopping, planning, etc.

that they disappear. I talked to my sister last night for the first time in several weeks—she's always flitting from one child to another—she has four, all grown—and it's often hard to locate her. I had hoped perhaps she'd decide to come here, had hoped she could just once make Stel's and my situation a priority—she knows how difficult it is—but no such luck. Six weeks in Germany with one daughter who is doing fine; four weeks in Seattle with another daughter who just had a second baby and is doing fine; two weeks with a son who just graduated from officers' training school; then a repeat of Seattle; a Thanksgiving visit with another son who is doing great in college—all of these things are priorities above coming here. She was here a week in the summer of '99 and it was a great help and comfort; has been through here for a day or two a couple of times since on her way to and from Germany, but no sustained visits. Ah, sorry to go on about this. I just find it hard to fathom why she (and various friends) can't set their priorities a little differently in the face of the dire circumstances we are dealing with here. For them, life just goes on as always and if they can't fit Stel and me into their normal busy schedules, then we lose out.

Actually, there is some positive news from the past few days. Stel's temperature has gone back to perfectly normal after being up and down and all over the place for several weeks. The doctor had decided the fever was probably disease-related rather than infection-related, but it appears to me now that that's not the case. She looks good, for someone who's been through what she has, and is doing well under the circumstances, but no improvement in responsiveness or functionality beyond being a little more awake on the Adderall. Re the Phosphatidyl, I started her on it and everything else you sent the day I got the package. No visible improvements as yet, but her situation is so severe, it may take more time if it is effective for her. I'm hoping anyway.

I feel better just from letting off some steam. Thanks for being a sounding board. Better get the day started. Kay

Mon Oct 30 2000 7:53 AM

Jeanne, I forgot to ask you about your comment that "there is often a REBOUND inflammation upon withdrawal of the Decadron." Could this account for much of the swelling on Stel's recent MRI, rather than tumor? She had been off Decadron just over four weeks. Kay

Thu Nov 02 2000 6:43 AM

Sharon, I just want you to know I'm emphathizing with you at this very difficult time. There are so many terrifying aspects about this disease but I think one of the most terrifying is how fast things can change. We constantly have to be prepared for another blow coming from a completely unexpected direction. I'm so sorry Daniel (and you) are going to have to go through more surgery, etc., but I admire your spirit. I'm following the same path—climbing any mountain and forging any stream to find ways to keep my beloved Stella from being robbed of her life. Kindest regards, Kay

Fri Nov 03 2000 9:03 PM

Dear Mr. [Gary] Reiss, I'm writing you at the suggestion of a friend about my partner Stella Sandris, who is suffering from a grade four brain tumor. Attached is a summary of her history over the past year. For the last several months, she sleeps most of the time; when she is awake, she's mostly staring off in space. Occasionally I can get eye contact with her and feel there is a connection there, but that has happened less and less in the last few weeks. She is unresponsive to any stimuli except for pain sometimes. The neurologist found her responsive when he pressed on her feet but not when he pressed on her hands. He said that she is in a stupor. Doctors are not sure why Stella is in this condition, given that her tumor has not been growing, but most think she is suffering from radiation injury, perhaps coupled with the effects of all the other traumas inflicted on her brain in the past year and a half.

Stella makes few sounds but sometimes grunts or moans if she's feeling some discomfort from some movement I'm making of her or, I assume, if she's passing gas or feeling some other pain (she has not experienced any significant pain that I'm aware of). On occasion, she has uttered small moans when I've talked to her that seemed like efforts to communicate, but that hasn't happened much lately. Sometimes she stares intently off into space and makes a noise as if she's startled or frightened. She also sometimes utters what sounds like "oh" when I'm feeding her through the tube, apparently indicating that her tummy's getting full. She clears her throat and sometimes coughs up mucus that troubles her. She is still able to chew and swallow fairly well if she's alert enough, which is seldom these days, except that the mucus seems to interfere with her swallowing sometimes. Her facial expression is mostly blank, but she does grimace and make very unpleasant faces when she's uncomfortable. She doesn't move any of her limbs voluntarily. Her right arm and hand are spastic and sometimes move involuntarily. Her left side is limp most of the time, but sometimes her arm or leg seems to have more muscle tone. I can move all of her limbs except her right arm easily and they are quite flexible. With some exercise, her right arm and hand become much easier to move as well. Despite all of this, Stella still has good color in her face, doesn't really look sick except for having no hair, and hasn't lost much weight.

I've tried various means of connecting with Stella. I talk to her a lot. I play songs that she knows well and sing them to her. I have audiotaped movies she is familiar with and TV programs I know she would be interested in and played them for her to listen to (I can't get the TV in a position where it might attract her attention and cause her to watch it; in the hospital I was able to do that a couple of months ago and she did seem to watch some programs. Now she seems much less able to focus, but I can't be sure because I don't have a way of putting the TV directly in her line of vision). I usually keep the radio or TV or music going in the room to provide some stimulus even when she seems to be sleeping soundly. I touch her and hug and kiss her and tell her I love her a lot.

Currently the neurologist is trying some medications to see if she will become more alert and responsive—stimulants and Parkinson's drugs. So far, she's been slightly more awake with the stimulant sometimes but there has been no other response.

I would like very much to talk to you about Stella's situation and whether the work you do with people in comas might be helpful to her. You can call me at just about any time of the day or night. I look forward to talking with you as soon as possible. The work you do gives me some hope that Stella can still be reached. Many thanks, Kay Loveland

Sun Nov 05 2000 2:55 PM

Kay—I think there are lots of possibilities for working with Stella, especially since there is no known physical reason for her to be in this state. At a minimum, we should be able to establish more communication. Also she stopped talking in June, which I consider a relatively short time ago in terms of these states. I will try to find time today to call; if not, I will be out of town until Tuesday and will call then. Thanks, Gary Reiss

Mon Nov 06 2000 7:40 PM

Dr. F: Did you have a chance to look at Stel's recent MRI that I sent down last week?

Tue Nov 07 2000 7:36 AM

[From Dr. Friedman]: Looks like more enhancing abnormality—I believe this to be tumor. Henry

Tue Nov 07 2000 10:34 PM

Dear Kay, I'm thinking of you and hoping there is some improvement for Stel. I have noticed A LOT of posts re the bad effects of WBR. Wish we had all known then what we know now so we could have made a more informed decision. But there will always be medical "misconceptions" (I didn't really want to use the word "mistakes") on the way to improved treatment options. Knowledge builds on knowledge. I know Steve's and Stella's doctors thought they were doing the best for them, at the time. They just didn't know ENOUGH. It doesn't help to get angry. However, I'm glad this issue is so much in the forefront on the List, because maybe our experiences with WBR will help those who haven't gotten to that choice point yet in their treatment. I'm doing okay—just managing, that's all. Miss Steve too much to feel anything but empty, for now. Take care of yourself and Stel. You're doing a fantastic job! Phyllis

Wed Nov 08 2000 10:50 PM

[To BT List]: Is anyone taking cyclophosamide (not sure of spelling) or know anything about it? Stel's oncologist says it's an anti-angiogenesis/chemo that is given in a low dose every day and doesn't have a lot of side effects. Dr. Friedman and she have suggested it for Stel. I've never heard of anyone taking it and would be interested in anyone's experience or information about it. Thanks, Kay

Wed Nov 08 2000 11:11 PM

Dear Phyllis, Thanks for your thoughts. Unfortunately, I can't report any improvement. We're adjusting meds, but nothing much has happened. I'm looking into a group who work with people in comas and minimally responsive states and are often able to bring them out of it. I may try it.

I'm glad, too, that more is coming out about radiation damage problems. People need to be aware of the risks.

I know how much you must miss Steve. I miss Stel every day and anticipate how much more I'll miss her if and when I can't touch her and see her beautiful eyes sometimes. I guess all we can do is let time take its course and, hopefully, assuage some of the pain. Take care of yourself. Kay

Fri Nov 10 2000 7:56 AM

Carol, Thanks for the message. Stel is back in the hospital as of yesterday morning. Emergency room doctors and surgeon and oncologist were giving me all kinds of dire predictions yesterday, but Stel is still ticking along today despite their best efforts to kill her off. Fortunately, my sister came to town night before last and was with me all day yesterday, so she had a chance to witness what I have to go through with these doctors, all of whom I think committed malpractice yesterday by not recommending a well-known medication for brain swelling, which I ultimately had to request, after I got my wits about me enough to remember it existed. Stel apparently has an infection that came on very suddenly that we don't yet know the origins of—maybe the IV line. There's also a lot of brain swelling, which we knew about more than two weeks ago with the MRI. The surgeon insists it's due to the fact that the tumor has grown so fast that it's now wrapping around the ventricles, etc. and there's nothing to be done. Strange that the doctor at Duke didn't have any such dire things to say about how it looked—or the neurologist. Maybe she's right, but I really believe I would be seeing changes in Stel I haven't seen during these weeks. In fact, until yesterday she was doing great in terms of temperature, infections, holding her own in every way. My sister thought the doctors were nuts—I'm glad I have a witness to it all. No one would believe it. I don't know what will happen next. If the doctors are right, Stel won't make it through all this. But she seems to be doing fine this morning. Kay

Sun Nov 12 2000 10:38 am

Dear Dr. Torres-Trejo, I sent Stella's latest MRI, done 10/24, to you last week and you should have it on Monday, the 13th. I would very much appreciate hearing back from you as soon as possible regarding your reading of it. Stella's surgeon has a very negative assessment—that the tumor has grown all around the ventricles and is obscuring them. I can't believe her apocalyptic vision because I haven't seen any significant changes in Stella over these past weeks. She's in the hospital now with a blood infection, and her breathing is not great, but she's holding her own, despite dire predictions by all doctors here. Henry Friedman, her neuro-oncologist, saw the scans and didn't have such dire things to say about them. I'd really like another view of it. I'll call you from the hospital late Monday or Tuesday and hope to talk to you about it very soon. Many thanks, Kay

Sun Nov 12 2000 11:01 AM

Friends, Stella is in the hospital. I took her to the emergency room on Thursday morning with a very high fever and high blood pressure and pulse. There was what I can only describe as near-panic by the ER doctors, who apparently thought she should already be long dead, given her diagnosis, and proceeded to tell me in the most extreme terms that she couldn't last long, especially given the swelling on her brain they saw on a CT scan. Her surgeon chimed in about the tumor growing out of control (despite lack of any clinical evidence of that in Stel's condition) and the oncologist bought it all, telling me she didn't think Stel could fight the infection and the brain swelling. Fortunately, my sister was with me and I had a witness to all this panic who thought it as wild as I did. After a day in the ER while her temperature came down substantially along with her blood pressure and pulse and she held her own, Stel was admitted to the hospital. She continued to tick along yesterday, with some breathing problems, and a temperature close to normal. They found she did indeed have a blood infection and she's on a variety of antibiotics.

There were more dire doctor's predictions last night by the oncologist's partner who thought her breathing indicated she couldn't go on much longer. She came through the night fine; her breathing is better this morning. It may be that the doctors are right, but I can't help but have my doubts, given the overreactions I've seen on several occasions over past months. I'm not sure at this point whether Stella may be slipping into a coma; she hasn't opened her eyes in the past few days, but she's been doped up with some morphine to help with breathing (she's not in pain). Unbeknownst to me, the nurses were giving it to her every two hours for some time before I got that discontinued, so I think she's still pretty sedated in addition to fighting the fever and infection, and that could account for her sleeping constantly. The next days will tell, I guess. I just don't know what to expect. I'm staying at the hospital around the clock, except for coming home this morning to do a few things. Please send all your most positive thoughts Stella's way. She's a real champ and confounding the doctors. Her surgeon said last night, "she's tough," and she's right. Kay

Mon Nov 13 2000 9:46 AM

Friends, With the deepest sadness of my life, I wanted to let you know that Stella died this morning, quietly and peacefully, without pain. I don't know as yet what funeral arrangements I will make. Please feel free to call me at home if you wish. Kay

Tue Nov 14 2000 6:18 PM

Dear Ms. Loveland: I have reviewed the MRIs from 10/24/00 and compared with the previous ones including 9/11/00. My impression is the following: The area of enhancement looks larger than previous MRI and surrounds the ventricles. One may think initially that perhaps this represents tumor more than anything else. I think that for most physicians the first thought is tumor because we want to be on the most cautious side for the benefit of the patient. I understand that Stella's neurological status has not changed which does not correspond with what we see in the MRI, although areas of enhancement many times get larger without affecting the patient's clinical status substantially.

One test that may be helpful to elucidate what this enhancement means is perhaps doing another PET scan but my feeling is that it may not show anything different from the previous PET done which, as you know, shows viable tumor. My impression is that the larger area of enhancement on this MRI most likely represents viable tumor.

I think at this point we need to define what to do next. I have the outline of what treatments she has had but please let me know what she is on right now regarding treatment for the tumor so I can suggest or think about other options. Please get in touch with me as soon as you can. Dr. Torres-Trejo

Wed Nov 15 2000 9:18 AM

Dear Dr. Torres-Trejo, Thank you for your reply. I am deeply saddened to tell you that Stella died two days ago. I had to take her to the ER last Thursday because of a 107-degree temperature and very high blood pressure and pulse. They found that she had a blood infection, probably from the IV line. She seemed to be responding well to the antibiotics over the next day or two. However, her surgeon was of the opinion that the tumor had grown substantially and enveloped the ventricles (a CT scan showed a great deal of swelling, as did the

MRI from late October). It appeared that the pressure on her brain adversely affected her respiration. She died peacefully and without pain.

I wish we had been able to consult with you much earlier because I believe she might, at least, have had some quality of life in this past year had she been treated at a major BT center by caring doctors like yourself who didn't look at her as an already dead person because of her diagnosis. Although we did consult with Duke, it was not close enough to have the kind of attention she needed. It is an irony of fate that we lived so long in Los Angeles (Stella was a graduate of UCLA) but were no longer there when this terrible illness struck. How fervently I hope that there will soon be a breakthrough in the treatment of this horrifying disease that will end the overwhelming suffering it causes to patients and caregivers. Thank you so much for your caring attention to Stella's case. Kay

Wed Nov 15 2000 10:05 AM

Dear friends [on BT List], With a heavy heart I write to tell you that my beloved Stella died at 4 a.m. on November 13th. She had been in the hospital for four days with a blood infection, which seemed to be responding to antibiotics. A CT scan showed extensive swelling and her surgeon said the tumor had grown substantially and enveloped the ventricles. I think the pressure on her brain ultimately made it impossible for her to breathe. I am grateful that her death was peaceful and without pain. About a minute before she drew her last breath, I had crawled into bed beside her.

Her valiant struggle lasted almost nineteen months, and the day before she died her surgeon looked at her with admiration and said, "She's tough." That same day a hospital attendant looked at her and said, "She doesn't look sick." She still had beautiful color in her face, which had hardly a line in it.

Stel was the most honest, self-aware, and emotionally trustworthy of people, the greatest, most loyal of friends, and a lively, intelligent, loving companion. I am a better, deeper person for having known her. Her life from childhood was never easy; she never got the recognition or rewards she deserved; fate pursued her to the end. But she had remarkable resilience, a great heart and soul, deep empathy and sensitivity for the less fortunate, and a feminist spirit from her youngest days. Most of all, she had an unbounded generosity of spirit; she was always more interested in helping, encouraging, and inspiring her friends in their lives and work than in advancing herself; whatever good fortune she had, which was precious little, she always wanted to share with others.

There is much, much more I could tell you about this wonderful woman who graced my life for 31 years. She was my heart and soul and I will carry her with me always. I don't know how I will get through so many days to come without hearing her melodious voice and her infectious laugh, seeing her beautiful golden brown sparkling eyes, feeling her soft, warm touch. But I was blessed that she loved me and chose to spend more than half her life with me. I won't see her like again. Kay

Index

A

Accutane 182, 199, 201, 206, 208
Acidophilus 81
Adderall 204, 208, 209
Akinetic mutism 134, 137, 144, 148, 157, 159, 168, 188, 189
Alternative treatments (Mexico, report, book) x, xii
Amantadine hydrochloride 156
Ambulance (long distance) 68, 183, 191
American Metabolic Institute (AMI) 67, 68, 75, 82, 83, 158, 178, 185, 187, 201, 204, 205, 206
Amino acids 105, 180
Anti-Alzheimer's medicines (see Aricept)
Anti-angiogenesis. (see Thalidomide)
Anti-coagulants. (see Heparin, Warfarin)
Anti-depressants. (see Effexor, Paxil, Zoloft)
Anti-Parkinsons medicines 159, 166
Anti-psychotic medicines. (see Risperdal)
Anti-seizure medicines. (see Depakote, Dilantin, Tegretol)
Apathy 48, 49, 51, 52, 137, 157, 194
Argenine 105
Aricept 156, 161, 168, 172, 174, 175, 178, 179, 181, 185

B

B-12 shots 131
Balance. (see Walking and Balance)
BCNU xii, 26, 32, 33, 36, 41, 42
Bending (at waist) 84
Bergsneider, Dr. Marvin 149, 153

Black, Dr. Keith 73, 87
Blisters. (see Sores)
Block, Dr. Keith 19, 34
   Natural killer cell blood test 31
Boots (protective) 80
Brain regeneration 54, 162, 163, 178, 180, 183, 198
Brain Tumor (BT) List xii, xiv, xv, xvi, 24, 87, 90, 92, 122, 144, 156, 175, 176, 182, 187, 195, 196, 200, 212
Brem, Dr. Steven 122, 130, 131, 136
Bromocriptine x, 124, 138, 156, 160, 166, 173, 177
Burzynski treatment 26

C

Carbo Dopa 161, 162
Carboplatin 72, 77
CCNU x, 41, 42, 46, 47, 48, 49, 52, 61, 63, 65, 89, 92, 158, 182
Cellulitis 80
Chemosensitivity testing (of tumor) 35
Chemotherapy x, xii, 10, 11, 13, 16, 17, 18, 20, 28, 29, 32, 46, 69, 76, 124, 148, 163, 164, 173, 179, 182, 185, 203
   Low-dose 186
Chestnut, Dr. Randall 74
Chicago Institute of Neurosurgery & Neuroresearch. (see CINN)
Chlorophyll 47
Choices in Healing xii, 73
CINN 31, 33, 34, 50, 78, 197
Clonus 99, 100
Cogentin 156, 168

Cognitive deficits. (see Apathy, Confusion, Initiative, Lethargy, Perseveration, Speaking, Word-Finding Problems, Writing)

Cognitive improvement 47, 52, 54, 59, 60, 61, 62, 64, 65, 66, 67, 68, 76, 77, 78, 80, 112, 113, 114, 115, 118, 119, 131

Coma 165, 211, 212, 214

Confusion 39, 127, 139, 166

Consciousness 173, 184

Corpus callosum x, 131, 139

CPT-11 32, 36, 61

Craniotomy x, xi, 24, 25, 90

Cyclophosamide 212

D

Decadron x, 14, 15, 25, 35, 36, 42, 46, 48, 73, 78, 101, 116, 120, 124, 129, 131, 138, 162, 196, 201, 202, 203, 208, 209

Dementia 131, 166, 172, 195, 196

Depakote x, 42, 60, 64, 65, 77, 110, 202

Dexamethasone. (see Decadron)

Diarrhea 81, 82

Dilantin x, 12, 76, 162

Dopamine agonists 134, 156, 159, 160, 173, 178, 179

Doppler blood flow study, cranial exam 134

Duke University. (see Dr. Henry Friedman, Dr. Leslie Forman, Dr. Renee Dunn, Bebe Guill)

Dunn, Dr. Renee 162, 174

E

Edema. (see Swelling)

EEG 40, 50, 60, 85

Effexor 161, 162

Enhancement. (see MRI)

Ephedrine 156

Epilepsy 162

Epileptologist 85

Exuderm bandage 79

F

Family and Medical Leave Act xi

Family Friendly Leave Act xi, 64, 93

Federal donated annual leave xi, 29, 58, 64

Fight for Life 67

Fine, Dr. Howard 128, 137, 139, 171

Forman, Dr. Leslie 162, 166, 168, 176

Friedman, Dr. Alan 168

Friedman, Dr. Henry xiii, 32, 33, 34, 41, 42, 47, 48, 49, 50, 52, 61, 65, 67, 93, 94, 129, 133, 137, 140, 148, 150, 154, 155, 156, 157, 161, 167, 171, 172, 177, 181, 182, 195, 198, 199, 201, 207, 212, 213

Frontal lobe x, 1, 4, 24, 32, 67, 73, 139, 153

G

Gait disturbance. (see Walking)

Gamma knife 21, 78, 195

Gliadel (chemo) wafers 35

Grossman, Dr. Stuart (Hopkins neuro-oncologist) 28, 31, 32, 33, 34, 41

Guill, Bebe 174

H

hCRF 124

Health Resource, The xii

Helenowski, Dr. Tomasz 33, 34, 36, 76, 78

Hematomas, subdural 142

Heparin 156, 168

Home assistance 46, 47, 49, 53, 55, 56, 58, 59, 79, 144

Hospice xiv, 53, 67, 72, 73, 86, 151, 159, 163, 164, 165, 170, 175, 178, 183, 184, 194, 201, 204

Hydragine 105, 117

Hydrazine sulfate 26

Hydrocephalus (fluid on brain) 104, 105, 106, 108, 117, 119, 120, 122, 123, 124, 126, 128, 129, 130, 131, 136, 137, 138, 139, 142, 143,

144, 145, 148, 150, 153, 157, 158, 163, 175, 187

   Normal-pressure 124, 138, 139, 141, 142, 148, 149, 157, 158

   UCLA program 139, 140, 141, 142, 145, 149, 153

Hyperbaric oxygen (HBOT) 131, 133, 134, 166, 176, 179, 194, 195

Hypermetabolism 156

I

Immunotherapy 37

Incontinence 52, 125, 137, 138, 139, 157, 166

Initiative (Motivation), lack of 37, 38, 39, 40, 48, 51, 52, 125, 128, 163

J

Johns Hopkins. (see also Dr. Stuart Grossman) 27, 28, 29, 30, 32, 33, 34, 36, 47, 141, 169, 182, 190

K

Kobrine, Dr. Arthur (Stel's first neurosurgeon) 2, 8, 10, 20, 23, 24, 25, 29

L

Lasix 70, 71, 208

L-Dopa (see Carbo Dopa)

Leaning, left, right 158

Lecithin 180

Lerner, Michael xii, 73

Lethargy 48, 51, 58, 87, 94, 98, 99, 112, 119, 120, 128, 165, 167, 195

M

M.D. Anderson. (see Dr. Christina Meyers)

Mannitol 96, 99

Marimastat 26

Medicaid 183, 184

Medical College of Virginia. (see Dr. Randall Merchant)

Melatonin 26

Merchant, Dr. Randall 32, 33, 35, 41

Metabolic causes, problems 76, 77, 197

Methotrexate 72

Methylphenidate. (see Ritalin)

Methylprednisolone 70, 71, 78

Mexico x, xi, xvi, 46, 83, 86, 87, 88, 89, 91, 92, 93, 95, 123, 125, 127, 128, 129, 135, 142, 143, 144, 157, 158, 159, 161, 169, 185, 193, 201, 204

Mexico journal 95– 121

Meyers, Dr. Christina xii, 125, 130, 131, 134, 171, 172, 173, 174, 175, 177, 179, 181, 185

Modafinil. (see also Provigil) 125, 185

Moss, Ralph, Ph.D xii

MRI

   Enhancement, Swelling 24, 25, 30, 32, 86, 87, 124, 209, 215

MRSpectroscopy 123, 133, 138

Mucus, in throat 170, 189, 210

Musella Website. (see Virtual Trials)

N

National Cancer Institute xii, 137

National Institutes of Health (NIH) 128, 139, 171, 190

National Rehabilitation Hospital 22, 46, 61, 63, 64, 65, 66, 74

Neglect. (see Weakness)

Neiman, Dr. Melissa (Stel's second neurosurgeon) 20, 21, 25, 121, 136, 152, 182

Neurontin 202

Neuro-psychologist, psychiatrist 41, 56, 76, 77, 157, 162, 163, 166, 171, 172, 174, 182, 183, 194

Nutritionist. (see Jeanne Wallace)

Nystatin 81

O

Oregon Health Sciences University 74

P

Pain 58, 210, 214, 215, 216

Paralysis 81, 90, 165

Paranoia 166

Paxil x, 134

PCV xii, 16, 26, 32, 33, 36

Peacock machine 32, 33, 34, 36, 78

Pentoxyfilline (Trental) 156

Perseveration 51, 157

Pessimism (of doctors) xiii, xiv, 64, 66, 135, 136, 146, 147, 148, 149, 150, 151, 163, 164, 165, 167, 168, 200, 203, 204, 216

PET scan 140, 141, 143, 146, 150, 155, 156, 198, 199, 215

Phosphatidycholine (PhosChol) 105, 180, 209

Physostigmine 156

Podiatrist 80

Poly ICLC 26, 32, 33, 35, 41

Poly-MVA 26, 101, 105, 107, 169, 178, 186, 201

Potassium 70, 71, 208

Prevacid x

Prolopa 156, 168

Provigil. (see also Modafinil) x, 156, 161, 166, 168, 178, 191, 192

Psycho-pharmacologist 135, 163

R

Radiation damage, injury, necrosis 130, 131, 132, 133, 134, 137, 140, 145, 147, 155, 156, 158, 159, 162, 163, 164, 166, 171, 174, 175, 176, 178, 179, 180, 185, 187, 189, 190, 191, 192, 193, 194, 195, 196, 197, 198, 199, 202, 207, 210, 212

Radiation treatment (standard) x, xi, xiv, 10, 11, 13, 14, 16, 17, 18, 19, 21, 24, 25, 43

　Effects of xiv, 14, 15, 16, 17, 18, 70, 76, 96, 130, 162, 163, 166, 175, 176, 192, 195, 196, 197, 210, 211, 212

　Low-dose 96, 97, 98, 99, 101, 108, 111, 186

Radioactive pellets 35

Rajagopal, Dr. Chitra 136

Rehabilitation 22, 23, 26, 56, 57, 58, 59, 60, 61, 62, 63, 64, 65, 66, 72, 74, 90, 157

Reiss, Gary 210, 211

Reiter, Dr. Joel 162

Requip 161, 162

Respite care. (see Home Assistance)

Retraining Cognition 66

Richard, Adrienne 162

Rigidity 101, 102, 119

Risperdal 166, 175, 176, 193

Ritalin (Methylphenidate) x, 59, 60, 65, 76, 77, 82, 124, 125, 129, 130, 131, 132, 133, 134, 135, 137, 138, 142, 159, 161, 164, 166, 168, 171, 172, 173, 174, 177, 179, 181, 185, 188, 191, 202, 203, 204

Rodakem 104, 105, 117

Rubio, Dr. Geranimo 87, 88, 96, 97, 99, 100, 101, 103, 104, 105, 106, 107, 108, 109, 110, 111, 112, 113, 114, 115, 116, 117, 118, 119, 120, 121, 178, 186, 187, 205

S

Seizures 20, 25, 36, 37, 40, 42, 43, 44, 50, 60, 62, 77, 82, 85, 96, 124, 128, 130, 131, 132, 137, 162, 173, 188

Selker, Dr. Robert 28, 35

Shunt x, 27, 106, 122, 123, 124, 126, 128, 131, 133, 135, 136, 137, 138, 139, 142, 145, 146, 147, 149, 150, 152, 153, 155, 159, 160, 162, 166, 167, 168, 169, 170, 172, 181, 182, 187, 188, 191, 193, 203, 206

Sores 79, 80, 110

Spasticity 102, 128, 129, 158, 211

Speaking 51, 52, 59, 60, 69, 71, 76, 77, 78, 79, 81, 82, 83, 97, 98, 99, 100, 101, 102, 103, 104, 105, 106, 107, 108, 109, 110, 111, 112, 113, 114, 115, 116, 117, 118, 119, 120, 121, 126, 127, 128, 142, 158

SPECT scan. (see MRspectroscopy)

Spells, right-sided rigidity 100, 101, 102, 103, 104, 105, 106, 107, 108, 109, 110, 111, 113, 114, 115, 116, 117, 118, 129

Spence, Dr. Alex 70

Spironolactone 70

Spontaneous Healing 8

Steenblock, Dr. David 133, 134

Stereotactic radiosurgery (one shot) x, xii, 28, 30, 31, 32, 33, 34, 36, 37, 38, 39, 40, 41, 42, 43, 45, 48, 49, 50, 51, 52, 53, 76, 78, 79, 88, 89, 157, 192, 197, 207

   Fractionated 78

Steroids. (see Decadron)

Stroke medicines 156

SU101 26

Sulci 130

Supplements. (see Vitamin/Herbal Supplements)

Surviving 'Terminal' Cancer xv

Survivors, long-term. (see also Ben Williams) xii, xv, 200

Swelling, brain. (see also MRI) 20, 25, 40, 42, 56, 86, 87, 120, 122, 123, 124, 127, 128, 130, 153, 201, 202, 209, 213, 214

Swollen ankles, glands 45, 49, 55, 79, 80, 81

T

Tamoxifen 26, 206, 208

Tegretol x, 12, 42, 60, 112, 172, 173, 188

Temodar (Temozolomide) x, 39, 41, 42, 61, 65, 68, 74, 75, 76, 77, 78, 79, 83, 88, 89, 92, 158, 163, 164, 201, 206, 208

Thalidomide 26, 32, 33, 167

Therapy

   Occupational and Physical vii, x, 14, 17, 18, 19, 22, 23, 26, 37, 47, 48, 51, 56, 61, 62, 63, 64, 65, 66, 68, 72, 74, 79, 90, 102, 142, 163

   Speech (Cognitive) x, 41, 47, 51, 52, 66, 74, 82, 83

Tijuana clinics 72, 73, 74, 75, 87, 88, 89, 92, 93, 94, 95, 96, 97, 98, 99, 100, 101, 102,

103, 104, 105, 106, 107, 108, 109, 110, 111, 112, 113, 114, 115, 116, 117, 118, 119, 120, 121

Torres-Trejo, Dr. Alejandro xiii, 187, 188, 198, 204, 213, 215

Transderm patch 170

Tremors 85, 115, 116, 202

Trental 156

U

UCLA. (see Dr. Alejandro Torres-Trejo, Dr. Marvin Bergsneider, Hydrocephalus)

Uncommunicative, unresponsive. (see Apathy, Lethargy)

V

Vaccine shots, therapy (Mexico) xi, 87, 91, 92, 93, 94, 96, 103, 104, 108, 109, 110, 111, 113, 116, 117, 118, 119, 120, 125, 127, 129, 135, 142, 158, 185, 186, 187, 201, 203, 204, 205

Ventricles 109, 122, 137, 139, 158, 172, 200, 203, 206, 213, 215, 216

Ventriculomegy. (see Hydrocephalus)

Virtual Trials (Musella) Website xii, xv

Vitamin/herbal supplements 47, 202

   Boswellin 202

   Bromelain 190, 202

   Selenium plus E 19

VP-16 94

W

Walking and balance (gait disturbance) 37, 40, 41, 42, 46, 48, 50, 51, 52, 56, 57, 61, 65, 78, 138, 153, 157

   Fast, leaning forward 110, 138, 143

   Improvement 36, 62, 63, 78, 83

   Leaning backward 36, 138

Wallace, Jeanne (nutritionist) 26, 31, 49, 52, 178, 190, 194, 207, 208, 209

Warfarin 156, 168

Weakness, overall 25, 32, 44, 71, 85, 136, 163, 166, 175, 196
   left-sided 44
   neglect 74
Weil, Dr. Andrew 8
White matter changes 122, 123, 124, 127, 128, 129, 137, 146, 150, 153, 158, 199
Williams, Ben xv

Word-finding problems 37, 38, 39, 40, 51, 52, 76, 77, 78
Writing 41, 51, 52

Z

Zantac x
Zofran x
Zoloft 134, 162

0-595-31960-2